Flying Under The Weather

Flying Under The Weather

Anecdotes from Fourteen Years of Practicing Aviation Medicine

JOHN A. SHEWMAKER DO

Copyright © 2016 John A. Shewmaker DO
All rights reserved.

ISBN-13: 9781530070404
ISBN-10: 1530070406

Table of Contents

Introduction ix
Ground School xi

Chapter 1 Really? No...*Really?*; or, You Can't Legally Fly
When You Pull the Wool Over Your Own Eyes 1
Chapter 2 No...Not Really; or, the Importance of Small Pauses. . . .8
Chapter 3 LateLiarEnglish™; or, I Said What I Thought
You Wanted to Hear but Meant What I Really
Wanted to Say 17
Chapter 4 Framing the Discussion; or, the Myth That the
FAA Process Is Onerous. 22
Chapter 5 Math and Myth; or, but I Saw It on the Internet so
It Must Be True 27
Chapter 6 Yet More Myths of the Third-Class Medical; or,
Trust Me, This Isn't Alzheimer's, My Keys Are in
the Goat!. 32
Chapter 7 Miscellaneous Anecdotes that Belong Somewhere;
or, Doesn't Everyone Else Throw Junk in a Junk
Drawer?. 37
Chapter 8 Beyond Judgment; or, I Don't Think They
Planned to Be Sociopaths, but That's
Where the Path Led 44
Chapter 9 And *You* Want to Fly *My* Airplane?; or, Is It
Easier to Go to New York or by Train? 53

Chapter 10	First-Time Problems; or, Why You Shouldn't Pretend Your Flight Doctor Is as Dumb as You've Heard............................66
Chapter 11	The Light Casualty Class of Aircraft; or, Why Can Grandpa Fly His Cub When He Can't Tie My Shoe?......................78
Chapter 12	What If You Commit a Crime and No One Wants to Help?; or, Doc, You Are so Uncooperative—Don't You Want to Be Roommates in Federal Prison?..................81
Chapter 13	But This Isn't Judgment Day; or, Judgment? We Don't Need No Stinkin' Judgment!..............87
Chapter 14	Is That a Pet Peeve, or Are You Just Way Too Sensitive?; or, If You Hear It Enough, You'll Go Blind.................................96
Chapter 15	Assorted Red Flags; or, You Told Me a Lot and Didn't Say Anything at All....................100
Chapter 16	What Brings You to My Business Today, Doc?; or, Never Park Your Ice Cream Truck in My Lobby......104
Chapter 17	Dealing with the Feds; or, How I Hope Semmelweis Isn't Applauding Me at the Moment....107
Chapter 18	Rip Van Winkle; or, How Bad Decisions Are Like Freeze-Dried Dandelion Seeds..............122
Chapter 19	A Typical Pilot's Vision Exam; or, Read the Bottom Line.................................130
Chapter 20	Defending Yourself for Doing Things Right; or, Do I Really Have to Pick up *Another* Certified Letter?.....................131
Chapter 21	Complaints Are a Dime a Dozen and Solutions Are Out of Stock; or, Are You Just Going to Whine, or Are You Going to Buy Something?........144
Chapter 22	Obesity: The Weighty Issue Plaguing America; or, Exercise Is the Cure to Rationalization............152

Chapter 23	Bad Judgment Is a Medical Diagnosis; or, Many Pilots Live in a Veritable Fog of Made-up "Facts"..... 161
	Table of Cessna 172 Fatal Accidents that I Have Categorized as Medically Related, 2000-2016 time frame:................................ 167
Chapter 24	Retrospective Assessment of Medical Factors and Decision-Making in Light-Sport Aircraft Fatal Accidents; or, Why Incapacitation Is Hardly the Real Measure of Whether an Accident Is Medically Related............................. 169
	Table of NTSB Reports Regarding Fatal Light Sport Accidents with Probable Medical Causative Factors. 174

Epilogue....................................... 175

Introduction

This is a compilation of thoughts, anecdotes, and concepts relevant to my past fourteen years of being an aviation medical examiner (AME).

I have tried to redact any readily identifiable information. Thankfully, most of these events happen repeatedly, so even if you think you might be mentioned in one of these anecdotes, you can take heart in the fact that you are a crowd—not an individual.

If this book offends anyone other than those pilots who lie, coerce, and exercise bad judgment; the USCIS; or pilots who can't laugh at themselves and at their own made-up little mythologies, then I apologize.

I will stress here and repeatedly that my few stories about interactions with the FAA directly are rare, rather than common events. I have been very lucky to gain from past experience the wisdom to always attempt collegiality and to generate an atmosphere of working together toward a common goal.

It is inevitable that in a huge department of government, you will meet some folks who simply can't get that basic concept or who frequently have "moments" as we all have at times. I relate several anecdotes that occurred over a period of twelve years, not because of their regularity, but because I am hard-pressed to think of many other bad experiences I have had.

I would hope any of my suggestions, pie in the sky or otherwise, are met with an understanding that I don't pretend to have all the answers; neither do I understand all the nuances under which a particular department or branch is forced to work. I also don't pretend to have the former competence in English writing and grammar that I once possessed as a student under Lawrence Smith and Bernie Miller at Eastern Michigan University. (That was thirty years ago.)

I have been especially blessed to work with many excellent professionals at the FAA Medical Certification Division, particularly the Atlanta offices.

It is important to note clearly that any statements regarding aviation medicine are my personal opinions as a physician. I am in no way speaking for the FAA or as a spokesperson of the FAA when I espouse these opinions.

Many of the events that occur in the book are rare. Others happen almost daily.

Ground School

As part of becoming a licensed pilot, the FAA requires most pilots to pass a medical examination. These exams are performed by Aviation Medical Examiners, as defined by the FAA. The FAA appoints flight doctors who are not employees of the FAA and provides training to these doctors. There are three classes of medical exams. First-class exams are required for airline pilots, often by insurance companies. Second-class exams are required for all other pilots who are using their license for commercial purposes such as giving sightseeing flights, mapping, banner-towing, agriculture, etc. The third-class certificate is for people who mainly fly as a hobby.

This book describes my personal experiences in aviation medicine. The events are all real, although occasionally I have changed the disease if rare, so as not to expose the pilot's identity.

One set of pilots does not require an FAA medical to fly: the light-sport pilot. They deserve a chapter all to themselves. The FAA allows them to fly over your house with little more than a driver's license as evidence of medical competency.

Getting a medical for aviation in many ways requires its own ground school. You need to know some basic information prior to just going off to get your medical. For that reason, I came up with the most basic rules I could, because I am a person who appreciates simplicity.

My Three Rules and Why I Have Them

Having been an AME for fourteen years and currently averaging about 180 flight exams a month, I have learned a few tricks to make my life easier and to make things easier on pilots coming to get their flight physicals.

Significant medical, mental, and legal issues will often result in delays for pilots getting their medicals. For almost all other issues, however, pilots can help themselves if they follow the three basic rules I tell each pilot every time they see me. There is no confusion—every time, every visit, I make it a point to tell the pilots my three rules.

Rule one: Never ask me to do anything illegal.

As absurd as that sounds, it bears repeating. Never ask me to do anything illegal.

The act of coercing a flight doctor can take many forms; all are attempts to coerce the flight doctor into a fraudulent conspiracy. The most obvious attempt is asking the flight doctor not to tell the FAA about a medical issue. This request is usually preceded by some comical statement, such as:

- "Off the record, doc…"
- "Now that I have my medical, let me ask you a question…"
- "Now, don't tell them this, but…"

So, what happens in cases like these? Well, let's look at the statements individually.

"Off the record"—I am not a journalist; it is all on the record.

"Now that I have my medical"—The FAA can reject your medical after you have an exam. The fact you have your medical in your hand isn't relevant if you are flying illegally. If you fly illegally with a dishonest medical form, you have committed perjury, have violated aviation law, and are subject to a five-year jail sentence.

A smart doctor will try to protect you by advising you not to commit a crime. The moment that you mention a grounding condition, the FAA doctor can and should immediately inform you that that medical certificate you currently possess may not be valid. The doctor should also document this with the FAA, otherwise you face increased risks and penalties.

"Don't tell them, but"—The AME is "them," so you are in fact telling "them" when you tell the AME anything. Why would you think otherwise?

No issue justifies lying to the FAA anyway. The idea that you'd ask someone who barely knows you to commit a felony and to put his or her professional license, family income, and reputation into a toilet simply so that you can commit a rash of federal felonies is a bit of a character and judgment issue. If you don't see the problem here, maybe aviation isn't your best choice. People die when pilots display poor judgment. Judgement occurs in your brain, thus, judgment IS a medical condition. Too often people seem to miss this point, and when the NTSB states an accident was due to a judgment issue by the pilot, the casual reader doesn't connect the dots. The crash was a medically caused crash, because judgment is a medical condition.

Sometimes the coercion is in the form of a "buddy pass," an offer to go up in an airplane ride, or the mere act of calling you by your first name. But make no mistake, if you fall for the quid, expect the pro quo.

Rule two: Never come to an exam if you are sick.

This should be painfully obvious. It is about judgment and about legal liability—but it is also basic common sense.

Why would you assume that your infection—which you can spread to all the other pilots in the AME's office—is so special that you deserve special consideration? Also, why would you ever expect an AME to certify you to fly an aircraft on a day when you legally shouldn't be in an aircraft?

Just having a common cold isn't a safe condition to fly for several reasons. Stay home, and come get your medical when you are better. Additionally, you are putting other pilots at risk of losing income simply because you assume you are more special than everyone else is in the world. Ultimately, this is a judgment issue—and judgment is a medical condition.

Regarding the common cold or allergies, over-the-counter sedating antihistamines such as Benadryl are one of the most common drugs found in the blood of pilots after fatal crashes. If you shouldn't be flying, please don't ask me to give you a medical saying you are OK to fly that day.

Rule three: If you have a medical condition, let the flight doctor know as soon as possible.

Handle paperwork issues well in advance of your medical, so that when you come to the flight doctor's office, you already know that your issue has been handled appropriately. Many pilots show up with new medical issues but make no prior notification. This often delays them from flying.

You might ask why these are my three rules. I don't have a rule about showing up in a pink panda bear outfit, but then I've not seen this occur on a consistent basis and therefore that rule isn't needed.

These rules exist because they address the most common things pilots do that have a negative impact upon properly receiving their medical.

That bears repeating: these are the most common actions that pilots take that can cause them to not get a medical on the day they have their exam. Frankly, that statement should scare you, because some of the folks who share our airspace—but not necessarily our judgment and competency—violate these rules on a regular basis. These people want nothing more than to fly on just a driver's license overseen by a DMV that no one on the planet thinks does an adequate job of screening drivers.

Using these rules will keep you from having many issues during your flight exam.

1

Really? No...*Really?*

or, You Can't Legally Fly When You Pull the Wool Over Your Own Eyes

THE NUMBER OF times a guy will try to fake his way through an exam and end up getting caught red-handed is baffling. You'd think that with a community of rumor-spreaders like the pilot clique, sooner or later the pilots would stop this nonsense. It hasn't happened yet, nor has it decreased in frequency.

Deception is a daily event, and if you only watch for it, you get better and better at finding it. Sometimes it is uncanny, because I won't even know what the red flag was, but for some reason I'll be picking up on a subtlety and *bam!* A second later, I catch a pilot in a bluff or a lie. I'd say that happens at least once a week.

▲ ▲ ▲

One day, a pilot walked in, strutted right into the exam room, and looked at the eye chart.

"D-E-F-P-O-T-E-C," he said, one letter after the other, crisp and sharp. It was so strange...almost as if he had memorized it letter for letter.

Pretty good vision, eh? It isn't like that isn't in several movies or anything. But we all know what this guy was up to. So, time to burst this poorly executed bubble. Instead of making him read line eight (the 20/40 line at my office), I decided to see how his 20/80 vision was.

"Very good, sir. Now read line four," I asked blandly. He proceeded to get it half right. "OK, then how about line six?" He got it all wrong except for two.

"Now line seven, backward?" He missed them all. "Now line eight, backward?" He missed them all again. He didn't pass.

On a brighter note, he had an excellent memory; that much was clear. Hopefully he came back when he got his glasses, but I can't remember.

▲ ▲ ▲

The flip side is that occasionally pilots will want you to fail them. Legally, it is an issue, because insurance fraud isn't a good business plan. My favorite failure was the guy who was really tired all the time and came in gray as a ghost.

"What organ did they transplant?" I asked, and he almost fell over.

"How'd you know?"

"It isn't hard. You've got the look."

"Liver transplant. The meds are killing me, but my insurer won't accept my word that I can't fly anymore."

And that pilot isn't flying anymore.

▲ ▲ ▲

Another pilot said "Huh?" or "What?" for every sentence out of my mouth. Finally, I stood right next to his ear and say, "I think you need hearing aids!"

"You think I need *what*?"

Boom! My son fell off his chair in other room. I could hear him rolling on the floor and laughing…but it wasn't like the patient could hear him. I didn't even lecture my son later on behaving professionally.

▲ ▲ ▲

This isn't even a hearing story, but another pilot wrote on a sign after his exam, "Why did I fail?"

He drove up to my office in a motor home, came in, and couldn't pass the *extremely* liberal vision test for a third-class medical. He was already stone-cold deaf, and his previous medical stated that he shouldn't fly anywhere he'd have to hear anything. (I may have paraphrased.)

He wasn't just deaf, he was also visually impaired. So on my sign, I wrote—rather small, since I do like to make my points clear—"You can't see."

"Can you write that bigger for me?" he wrote.

Later, his assistant called. It happened to be his home health aide, who assisted him daily because he found it hard to function. The aide wanted to know why he had failed his exam!

I hold no illusions about being helpful to this gentleman; he has no business in the air, ever. In fact, he shouldn't have been allowed to fly when he was deaf, but no one ever votes for me when I run for king, so there it is.

▲ ▲ ▲

Another pilot never had a major issue but needed his ECG done as part of a minor surgery. I did it, and it had some new findings from previous ECGs.

He went off to his cardiologist, and the cardiologist called and told me, "John, I think the autoimmune disease has spread to his heart."

"What autoimmune disease?" I asked.

"Oh, I thought you knew."

Thunk, thunk, thunk, went my head.

▲ ▲ ▲

Pilots don't realize how easy it is for one aspect of the exam to go awry and suddenly their old medical issues come flooding out. Sadly, it often doesn't need to happen. If the pilot is honest and does not illegally fly with a known condition, usually they are able to fly on a special issuance document that the FAA uses to track pilots with known medical issues.

One day a pilot who appeared to be in his mid to late fifties and whom I have never met before, walked in. He was very pale. Casper the Friendly Ghost pale.

The first seven words out of this man's mouth rolled out as slowly as water forming a very tiny bubble that gradually builds to a larger bubble, then falls to the ground.

It was painful to listen to him as he said, "I…am…here…for…my…flight…exam."

I resisted the urge to say, "Oh, that was yesterday," because he wasn't going to get the joke. I knew he was anemic before we even thought about forms.

I asked him if he had been especially tired lately or noticed anything unusual in his bowel movements. Yep, he said he had been having some bleeding for several months, so I am thinking colon cancer pretty seriously. Naturally we didn't give him his medical, but sent him off to get diagnosed. Two months later, his wife sent me a Christmas card and he got all better. We got him a special issuance within months after his surgery for colon cancer. It isn't magic; it's probability.

Six years later, I got a phone call from another flight doctor. This gentleman is relatively new to the AME business, but we have known each other awhile. He wanted advice on how to handle a case regarding a previous history of colon cancer.

I asked him who did the last physical, and he said, "He doesn't know, some fat guy on Colonial."

Thunk, thunk, thunk.

"That was me! You are speaking to John ColonCancerGuy, aren't you?"

"Wow, you are good."

Thunk, thunk, thunk.

Turns out, the guy went to him to renew his medical after not getting it renewed for a couple of years; however, he couldn't remember my name. Of course, it was on the special-issuance letter in his hand because they also send it to the doctor who did the last exam. But he tells the other flight doctor he went to the fat guy on Colonial…

OK then.

▲ ▲ ▲

Another day, a gentleman took up the first fifteen minutes of his appointment to make sure he got his car properly aligned in his parking slot. Eventually he walked in, pale and not in the biggest of hurries. He had a lot of trouble hearing and seemed a bit confused by my questions. This pilot was clearly not able to make good, quick decisions and would be a definite risk to life and limb if he were to get into an airplane. I deferred his exam because he seemed to have a lot of confusion, and I felt he needed a full neurological evaluation.

An airplane assumes you will be competent.

He called later and told me, "Oh, I just get nervous when I go to have my flight exam."

Of course, it took him a bit of time to get that sentence out, and it was in a voice that made me wonder if he was in a helicopter. (He was not.) Kindly, I didn't remind him that he had fifteen minutes to calm down while he was backing into and out of my parking lot slots while snails passed his car. Outliers of nervous make me a nervous doctor.

The last I heard, he hadn't been granted a medical; although AOPA (Aircraft Owners and Pilots Association) would have no problem with him flying over schools with just his DMV license, despite him being nothing but a major threat to anyone in any form of transportation.

Later, his wife called and said, "We told him we don't think he should even be driving."

"Yeah, so?"

"But that would crush him."

"Only figuratively, lady. A semitruck will do it literally." I probably just thought it.

▲ ▲ ▲

Sometimes impatience will be a clear sign of a medical issue. A gentleman who had never been to my office had an 8:30 a.m. appointment. My office was inside a larger building with multiple offices. I was the first to arrive that morning. I was sitting in my car, waiting for the building to open. I saw a person walk up and check the door at 8:20 a.m., turn around, get in his car, and drive away.

The door was unlocked at 8:25 a.m. I entered to open my offices, and the phone rang.

"Are you guys there? I had an appointment at eight thirty."

"Yes, sir. I am in the office."

"Well, the doors were locked, so I left."

"You had an eight thirty appointment. When did you check the doors?"

"At eight twenty. You weren't there, so I left."

"Well, it is only eight twenty-eight. Come on back."

"It's too late. I have to go."

This told me that the gentleman was simply in too big of a rush to be honest when asked about his medical history, too big of a rush to fill out the forms, and so on.

That person doesn't belong in an airplane, because preflights aren't optional and this type of personality will think that they are.

▲ ▲ ▲

That reminds me of school physicals.

A mother asked me for advice about her morbidly obese six-year-old. I said, "Send him to college immediately."

"Huh?"

"Ma'am, your child is a stinking genius."

"Huh?"

"Ma'am, you have a kid who is morbidly obese. You obviously couldn't be the issue, or you'd say, 'Hey, doc, I think I'm addicted to overfeeding my child.' The school can't be the issue; they tell everyone they are competent professionals, as highly skilled as Louisa May Alcott was when she taught elementary school as a fifteen-year-old and was having a much better graduation rate than they. So there can be only one explanation: your child has figured out how to get a part-time job, hide it from you, stash his funds or convert them to a food that is invisible, and then eat it all. That can be the only reason he's gained too much weight."

She looked at me for a second and said, "Yeah, we probably do overfeed him."

Thunk, thunk, thunk.

Sometimes the cause of a problem simply doesn't recognize they are the cause of the problem. Might make a nice T-shirt to give to people, eh? If you know someone who is the cause of the problem, buy the shirt and pay me a royalty—4 percent seems fair. I can't wait to see all those CAUSE OF THE PROBLEM shirts walking around.

▲ ▲ ▲

Another day, a woman was cussing and yelling at her kids in the office, hence, we asked her to leave. She went off on a rant about it being a free country and how she can say anything she wants.

"You are correct," I said. "It is a free country…and you are free to get your butt out of my *not free* dictatorship of an office and walk around that free country outside all you like, being the absolute worst excuse of human being or parent that you want to be. In here, however, this is not a free country, and physicians can call the police and force you legally to stay locked up in a psych ward for three days, so if you are here for four more seconds, you are legally crazy. And you are now at three."

After all, what kind of sane person would sit in a doctor's office—who can legally commit them—after the doctor has told them to get out?

Get your CAUSE OF THE PROBLEM shirts while they're hot!

▲ ▲ ▲

If the old saying is, "the early bird gets the worm," would it not make more sense to fill the birdfeeder with worms instead of birdseed? Or is it all about us, and the bird's taste is irrelevant?

2

No...Not Really

or, the Importance of Small Pauses

THERE'S ONE LINE I hear quite often that always catches my attention. When I hear it, I *always* dig in a bit. A pilot calls my office to schedule an appointment, and I ask if he or she has any medical issues.

And there it is: "No...not really."

The pause is the important thing. *Not really* said fast often turns up little things like cholesterol...but *No*...[slightest of pauses]...*not really* can be hiding a huge issue.

Take-home message: don't ignore being "no...not-really'ed."

▲▲▲

I saw a gentleman one day whom I had known for years. I asked, "Anything wrong since your last visit?"

"No...not really." But during his exam, the gentleman couldn't turn his head at all to the left.

"What's wrong?"

"Nothing, really. I just have to get this disc repaired soon, or it's gonna kill me."

"It should stand in line…"
He thanked me later after his surgery for properly doing his exam.

▲ ▲ ▲

Another pilot "no…not really'ed" me after a yearlong battle he was having with doctor wannabees committing malpractice on her.

This pilot mentioned on the history form that he had made seven visits to local minute-clinics for sinusitis infections over the past year. When I asked about his ENT (ear, nose and throat specialist) visits, however, he stated he hadn't been referred to a specialist.

Right away, I knew I'd find a "yes…yes really" problem, and so I put my otoscope into the patient's nostril. Well, no…not really; what I did was attempt to insert the otoscope, but the polyp that was poking almost out of the nostril completely prevented me from examining that nostril.

This person's experiences with people who wanted to be doctors but didn't want to go to medical school had led him to waste a year not being treated for an easily diagnosed medical condition. Meanwhile, he placed himself and passengers at risk by flying with a potentially devastating medical condition that could have immobilized him at a very bad phase of a flight descent.

Take-home message: if you think you are a Maserati, don't get your mechanical work done by your neighbor, Bob, who works on his Jeep every weekend.

▲ ▲ ▲

On polyps and "no…not really." Another gentleman brought in his CPAP machine data showing how well his sleep apnea was being treated, but he didn't have the required physician's report.

"Any other issues?"

"No, not really." Then he said, "Hey, wait! I think it's in the car." He went to his car and brought back an ENT letter that he tried to pass off as his sleep study report. This failed because the report he brought me instead is about an office visit for chronic sinusitis; he had nasal polyps.

He said, "Oh, yeah. I am getting surgery. Would have been sooner if my ENT wasn't on vacation."

I advised him that we needed more input regarding risk of sinus block as well as a better letter from his sleep specialist, and he got upset.

"I have to fly tomorrow," he wailed. Yet later in the conversation, he admitted to being congested.

Thunk, thunk, thunk goes my head on my desk. This is a pilot who doesn't get it.

▲ ▲ ▲

A pilot came in from the hot summer sun, and he was sweating.

"Any medical problems?" I asked.

"No...not really."

Then I noticed he was shivering and I asked him about it.

"Oh, my wife was really sick last week; now I think I have it."

And the Lysol cloud filled the air, and darkness was upon the face of the earth.

▲ ▲ ▲

A favorite:

"Do you have a primary care physician?"

"No...not really."

There are thousands of pilots who get zero preventative health care and who say such things as, "Oh, I feel great. Why would I go to a doctor?" These folks seek out the best mechanics in the world to work on their airplanes, but disconnect totally from the concept that *they* are the key cog on the airplane's equipment list.

And if you read NTSB fatal accident reports, you'll soon find that some don't bother with the best mechanics either.

▲ ▲ ▲

This raises important questions about the push to get rid of the flight medical by the sickest people in aviation. This isn't an accident; there is a group of pilots who will lie about their health, lie about medical histories, and lie about the FAA and flight doctors. These pilots are pushing legislation to get rid of the third-class medical, and their entire push is based upon myth.

Many pilots who are in perfect health have zero idea of the dozen pilots each month that I stop from getting a medical. Nor do they see the hundreds of other pilot applicants turned away from other AME offices. Even the healthy pilots who seriously believe that the third-class medical has no value don't grasp that healthy pilots over age sixty-five are at best a slim majority (and more likely a slim minority) of all third-class pilots, and their belief is built upon myth and wish, and not on one iota of reality.

In one typical week, I had a pilot whose doctor spilled the beans about his atrial fibrillation, a pilot who first stated he had zero medical problems and then claimed his mental illness was more severe than most people's, a person who falsified a medical exam date, a pilot who came to the exam quite ill, and a pilot who admitted he had left off significant issues on a previous exam. This wasn't atypical; in fact, this was a slow week.

▲ ▲ ▲

One of the best "no…not really" moments came when a gentleman called and asked for an appointment one day.

He started off with, "I am trying to get back into the air; it's been a while."

"Any medical problems?"

"Oh, not…[slightest of pauses]…not really."

"What medical issues have you had, sir?"

"Well, I did have a pacemaker and a defibrillator placed about twelve years ago, but I am all better now."

"So, how would you feel if you were landing at an airport where you have never landed, at two in the morning, forty feet in the air in a driving rain, crabbing into a crosswind of ten knots, when all of a sudden your defibrillator goes off?"

"Oh, I would never fly in those conditions!"

"And yet, people do fly under these conditions and die every month in just this scenario. That is probably why the FAA doesn't allow defibrillators in pilots." (Unless they are going light sport, but that is a bit of cynical inanity that I will discuss elsewhere.)

The last part of the dialogue was internal, as I likely only informed this potential applicant that the FAA didn't allow pilots to fly with defibrillators. I'm sure as I hung up, I reflected that I had blocked another potential applicant from placing himself into harm's way.

These are not rare conversations; they occur at my practice on the order of four or five people a week who have disqualifying conditions but who call about getting a medical. And they've been calling every week for the past twelve years. If you are doing the math, that means I have personally, hopefully, prevented about twenty-four hundred people from taking to the air when they had no business in an airplane.

▲▲▲

One of the earliest stories I have concerns a gentleman who walked in, dragging his left leg and left arm. So the conversation goes, "When did you have your stroke?"

"Twenty years ago."

"Are you a pilot?"

"Yep. Got two thousand hours."

"When was your last medical?"

"Oh, I never bothered; just figured I'd get legal now since I have been doing this for twenty years. And what the hell—I might want to get a bigger airplane. I might need more training."

▲ ▲ ▲

One great "no…not really" was the day a pilot said, "Oh, no…not really. Just a ministroke, but I'm all better." And this gentleman had continued flying, regularly.

I had known this third-class pilot for quite a few years, and for the first time since I'd known him, he brought in a stack of papers.

So I asked him, "You mean to say, you had a blood clot in your brain that temporarily caused parts of your brain to shut down?"

"Yep."

"And did the clot know which blood vessel to shut down, or did it just randomly pick one?"

"Uh, I dunno…"

"Never mind. Anyway, we need A, B, C, D, and E documents—"

"But I was gonna go flying this week!"

Thunk, thunk, thunk, goes my head on the desk. I continued explaining to him what documents he needed. Meanwhile, he denied any other issues or history of atrial fibrillation.

When his medical records arrived, it turned out that he not only had a long history of paroxysmal atrial fibrillation (a disease that makes a pilot more prone to throwing blood clots into his major arteries), he has also had *multiple* ministrokes and has lied to the FAA for, at the minimum, ten years.

This pilot, with a series of severe medical issues, had simply been going off to the airport and taking his family's and friends' lives into his hands with the mind-set of "oh, that will never happen to me."

So anyway, I looked at his MRI reports, and they showed multiple areas of damage—of strokes. Not TIAs (ministrokes). *Real strokes!*

I told him this, and he said, "Well, I never felt anything."

And I softly said, "It was likely in your judgment center. Those areas you don't feel it."

Judgment is a medical condition.

We sent all his paperwork in, but I explained to him that, not only would I not fly with him, I wouldn't let him drive me in a golf cart covered in bubble wrap…

Six weeks later, his certificate came in the mail. I just threw all my papers in the air and asked, "What is my purpose, if this guy gets a medical?" I was alone, so you'll have to take my word on it.

To cap it all off, he called and bragged about getting his medical and how he couldn't wait to take his wife and two kids on a flight. *Thunk, thunk, thunk,* went my head on the desk…and with a high degree of probability, so will his family.

▲ ▲ ▲

I have evidently told way too many of these stories over the years, because one day, a guy walked in, got to the exam room, and started telling me about his new heart valve.

I started huffing and puffing, and he said, "Aww, I am just messing with you. You taught me not to do that."

I didn't know if flattered or anger was the right feeling. At least he had remembered my warning.

He proudly walked into the lobby and said to everyone in earshot, "You should have seen his ears turn red. I got him good!"

I hope he reads this; he knows who he is. He's the one with severe halitosis that I have just slandered and immortalized simultaneously in this magnificent text. That is called payback.

▲ ▲ ▲

Paperwork can sometimes be presented as a "no…not really."

Often you need to check medical reports, and you learn to do it extremely carefully. (This is polite, subtle talk for: *Read every word of every report every time!*) Sometimes it is a third party that "no…not reallys" the pilot.

In this event, an airline pilot was told that his paperwork was good, when it actually had a major issue. This happens a lot with unnecessary third-party groups. This gentleman had a new onset history of atrial fibrillation earlier in the year. The guy told his third-party medical advisory group and they said, "Just take your paperwork to your next flight physical."

"Hey, doc. They are paid by my union. Just defer me, doc. They're handling everything."

Some airline unions and aviation groups have "medical experts" to help their pilots fly safely....some are quite good, while others....

None of them are as good a source of information as the qualified flight doctor who hits the "print certificate" button. For information about whether your flight doctor is going to print you a certificate, the smart money always goes to the source first, and doesn't waste time on third parties. And, thus, I explained this to the pilot.

"No problem," I said, "but let me explain the nuances of why you want the person who prints your certificate onboard..."

So we got all done, and he said, "Hey, I do see your point, so even though I really don't trust you—after all, you are a tiny doc-in-a-Box I've never seen and you are a bit odd and they are the big union doctors—I'll send you a copy so you can review it."

So I said, "Well, going forward, involve me early."

He left, and a couple of days later, he sent over a bunch of stuff. While reading his past medical history (where the lies of the past come back to haunt him) I find listed a stent placement. *Hmm*, he didn't say anything about that.

So I e-mailed him and asked, "Hey, when did you get stents in your heart?"

"I ain't never had stents. That must be a mistake."

I explained that the discrepancy could cause him a future medico-legal issue and that he should fix it by getting his treating physician to correct the error.

He does and then e-mailed back: "Of all the people who looked at my stuff, you are the only one to find it."

Yet, these tiny issues that have huge implications are the norm when it comes to the third parties. When a pilot is looking for 100 percent performance from the third party groups, being right 95 percent of the time just doesn't cut it. And the sad part is, the pilot usually gets mad at the flight doctor and has to be gently educated that it isn't the flight doctor who is the problem, it is the third party that doesn't realize "stent placement" is a bit of problem for the pilot.

If there is one truth to reviewing reports, it is this: *Read every word of every report every time!*

▲ ▲ ▲

Often the FAA finds out about past medical issues when a patient brings in medical records from a totally unrelated issue. A pilot might bring in reports for his hypertension and on page fifteen will be listed, "brain aneurysm" or "committed for involuntary three-day mental hold." These types of things happen about ten times a year in our practice, when a patient shows up with medical records after flying illegally for years with a serious medical issue. The AME requests Record A and ends up getting Record Hey! Wait a second!

Sadly, many pilots think nothing of flying with severe medical issues and will hide them—taking on the risk of a $250,000 fine and a five-year jail sentence. They also think nothing of placing at risk their family, friends, and people in the homes, cars, and schools below them on the ground.

In the older, third-class pilot community, this is likely either a majority or close to it. Sometimes a tangent is the only point on a circle.

3

LateLiarEnglish™

or, I Said What I Thought You Wanted to Hear but Meant What I Really Wanted to Say

People often make statements that are not the words they are using. For instance, they might say, "When is the latest appointment of the day?" In school and to concrete thinkers, this seems like a question.

It isn't a question.

When you consider that statements are processed ideas, not the actual idea itself, you realize with time and experience that some questions are actually statements.

The statement these people make when they ask "what is the last appointment of the day?" is: "No matter what words come out of your mouth next, I will be late. But I promise to call you one to three minutes before I am late to tell you I will be ten minutes late. I will actually be thirty minutes late, though."

When you understand this, the conversation then involves questions and statements where the questions aren't answered in a traditional manner. To an outside observer who only views *words* as honesty and not *ideas* as honesty, it will seem like the doctor or the patient is lying. In fact, it is simply a variation of a very honest form of sending ideas back and forth. So here is the scene:

Pilot: I need a flight physical; when is the last appointment of the day?
Me: Four thirty.
Pilot: I'll take it.
At precisely 4:28 p.m., the phone rings.
Me: Hello?
Pilot: Hi. I am running about five minutes late.
Me: OK, I'll wait until four forty-five. If you aren't here by then, I have to leave.
Pilot: Oh, well, it may be more like twenty minutes.
Me: All right, but I swear, if you show up at four fifty-one, you're wasting your time. I'll wave to you as I leave.
The actual conversation is far different from the verbal, English conversation. It goes:
Pilot: No matter what you say, I will be thirty minutes late
Me: So be here at five o'clock. I'll fit you in, and if you are late, I will do the five-thirty person before you. And don't you dare whine if I do.
Phone rings:
Pilot: I told you I would be thirty minutes late.
Me: I have no sympathy and will cancel you if you aren't here.
Pilot: OK, I've got to speed up. Be there in a second.
Me: Whatever.

And I booked her for a five o'clock appointment. So the pilot showed up at five o'clock for her four-thirty appointment (that I had already written down as five o'clock), and she didn't say a word when my five-thirty appointment showed up and says, "I am here for my five-thirty exam."

Not because she wasn't thinking, *Hey! He lied about that latest appointment,* but because she didn't know that I speak her duplicitous language. She didn't want me to say, "So what? You were thirty minutes late. I already had to cancel my stuff, and this guy called while I was sitting down twiddling my thumbs, waiting on you to drag your butt in here late again."

It was her shame at being late and not being able to argue with me that kept her from saying, "Hey, wait a second!" And I had zero guilt about that;

in fact, I kinda enjoy it, because if I didn't speak LateLiarEnglish™, I would have been there till 6:30 p.m., waiting for this self-absorbed, rude person to show up late, as she consistently does. It's all about the economics.

So, I always mark yes when asked if I speak a foreign language. I am fluent in LateLiarEnglish.

▲ ▲ ▲

One Saturday, a gentleman called at eleven to ask what time his online appointment with a confirmation e-mail was. (It was for three o'clock.)

Now, knowing he was going to be late for his three o'clock appointment, I told him noon.

He says, "OK, I'll see you soon."

I promptly moved his online appointment to twelve thirty, since I knew that was when he would be there. At twelve, he called and told me he was going to be late, so I yelled at him for being rude enough to think that I would still be waiting around for someone on my weekend. Then I hung up my phone and laughed. At twelve thirty we did his exam, and at one, my one o'clock pilot showed up. I went home at three instead of three thirty, because he had been the last appointment of the day, but his chronic inability to plan ahead had caused him to come in two hours early.

You have to work within the framework of what you have, not within the mythology of what you want the world to be.

And before you accuse me of lying, reconsider: the language we were using wasn't traditional English at all. That is the point—an idea is complete in the mind but incomplete in the expression. The ideas were pure.

Him: I am gonna be late.
Me: It isn't going to affect me.
Him: I told you I'd be late.
Me: So what?

That is the translated version of the very honest conversation. Any confusion is in the mind of the pilot solely because he thought he was the only one speaking his language. It isn't my fault if I speak clearly to you in your language and you don't recognize it.

That brings me to a new topic: foreign pilots. But I will weave that topic into other chapters.

▲ ▲ ▲

Drug users use a variation of LateLiarEnglish™ called "Why is this on your exam?"

A twenty-four-year-old walked in. I handed him a urine cup. He looked at it and then at me and said: "I didn't have to do this on the last exam!"

"When was that?" I asked.

"Five years ago."

Thunk, thunk, thunk.

"Well," I said, "then you have been flying totally illegally for the past five years, so you need to do it ASAP." (The joke went right over his head.)

The urine test has been a requirement for years, so maybe the last doc was ninety-three and forgot to do it…but what probably happened, based on how fast the pilot ran out of my office was he was a pot smoker. Just guessing.

▲ ▲ ▲

Some people call on the phone speaking a dialect of LateLiarEnglish™ that I call, DummieOnDrugsEnglish.

"What is all tested on the FAA exam?" They ask.

"Well, we test for all the drugs out there, hair samples for past use, all police records, and juvenile expunged files—"

Click, buzz.

So, how did the real conversation go, translated into English?

"Do you guys test me for drugs?"

"Just did it; you failed."

▲ ▲ ▲

Guy called and said, "I am going to be in Amsterdam next week, but the FAA wants me to send them a urine sample within five days, because of my last pot arrest."

▲ ▲ ▲

You can also test sketchy people by the non-drug-test drug test.

It goes like this: you send them into the restroom with a cup. When they come out, you go into the restroom and close the door. Then you sit there on the toilet with the seat down (because otherwise you would feel strange), and five minutes later, you come out and pull them aside. Then—and this is the most important part—you spend enough time acting like you are trying to think of how to ask them a question that you see a stress reaction in them…sweat beading on the forehead, lip biting, hand tapping. Then you say, "So, what did I find in your urine, buddy?" And they tell you! This is a very low cost drug screen.

The FAA doesn't actually require a drug test for an FAA medical, but if an applicant doesn't know it and seems sketchy, you might want to try using a non-drug-test drug test.

4

Framing the Discussion

or, the Myth That the FAA Process Is Onerous

MANY PEOPLE THINK that most back surgeries are failures. Actually, most back surgeries are highly successful. So, why do people think the surgery is risky and that it usually doesn't work?

Simple: because the 5 percent of patients with failed back surgeries complain loudly and often, but the 95 percent with successful back surgeries don't talk about it that much. In the same way, the angry, disgruntled (and often dishonest) pilot creates "truth" out of a total lie.

The FAA process is actually not that onerous, provided you don't have a medical issue that comes up within three months of your next exam, and provided you are proactive. As long as you are proactive and your medical issue isn't a major, life-threatening one, the FAA process is simple, easy, and well thought out. When pilots adhere to the following simple steps, 99 percent of the time, they will get through the process easily and without being overly burdened.

So what are these steps?

Step one: when you have a problem, don't listen to a third party. Don't pay a third party for help, and don't allow groups to take your money because they pretend they can help you get your medical faster. The truth is that they are slower. They often give incorrect information, and at the end of the day, if they say one thing and the AME says something different, you are going to be unhappy.

Step two: call the AME quickly, and don't wait until the exam is due. The AME is the person who will give you your medical; you want the AME's opinion early, so that you can gather all necessary information and give that information to the decision-makers, not the third-party groups pretending to be your advocate while charging you exorbitant fees for services your AME should be able to handle.

Besides, one way to really upset an AME is to expect us to dig through three hundred pages of records on the day of your visit. It doesn't just upset our schedule, and it isn't just rude. It's also a recipe for disaster, since it could result in your exam being deferred.

Step three: don't exaggerate and don't overstate. Suppress the need to explain yourself and instead listen carefully to the steps the AME gives you.

Following these three steps will eliminate the majority of problems a pilot will ever have with the FAA from a medical issue. Not following these steps virtually guarantees that you will have at minimum a minor delay in getting your medical, and you will possibly become upset and have a major delay. Why? Well, that is what I am going to demonstrate with some hypothetical examples.

▲ ▲ ▲

One early January morning, Joe A. Rrythmia is diagnosed with premature ventricular contractions on an exam at his personal doctor's office. He has a full work-up, and his doctor tells him he is perfectly fine and that he had nothing to worry about. Relieved, Joe goes about flying his 172 over the local IHOP to impress the locals. Six months later, he shows up to get his flight exam, knowing he is at the peak of fitness as a thirty-two-year-old, successful sausage manufacturer. On his MedXPress form, he mentions a visit to his health professional, citing only a cardiac problem.

The AME asks him what the problem was, and Joe states, "I dunno, some type of arrhythmia, the nurse said, but I am fine; they did a full work-up on me." The AME asks for additional medical records, and immediately Joe starts getting upset and defensive: "Hey, I am fine. I had a full work-up—why do I need to give you any records?"

Six weeks later, the FAA finally clears Joe because the AME doesn't have time to waste getting into a personality conflict. Joe spends the next six months whining about how evil, onerous, and bad the FAA is and how they don't want to help pilots. All of this was totally avoidable, but because Joe is the local IHOP legend, he is believed by all…and the dishonest myth is spread.

So what would have been a better approach?

Joe should call the AME immediately following his personal doctor's diagnosis and tell the AME he's been diagnosed with an arrhythmia. The AME then tells him to e-mail him all his records after he has a full work-up. Joe does so, and the AME forwards this benign condition to the FAA. The FAA sends Joe a letter clearing him to fly. Joe goes to his exam, the AME tells him "great job," and the world is a better place. A few flowers even start blooming.

This example shows how one pilot's arrogance, lack of foresight, and sensitive ego manages to create a totally false mythology about the process of getting a medical.

▲ ▲ ▲

Patrick Picksalot experiences a nosebleed that won't stop. He uses a piece of toilet paper every hour, but the slow drip-drip-drip every fifteen seconds finally irritates him enough that he drives forty miles to the ER. He walks in at 4:00 p.m. with the complaint that his nose is slowly dripping blood, and he is getting a bit tired of it. The ER doctor asks if he has any other problems, and Patrick says, "Yeah, hemochromatosis; nothing else." The ER staff then treats Patrick with Neo-Synephrine, and a friendly nurse presses his nostrils together for five minutes. Packing is placed, the doctor tells him to skip next month's visit to the Red Cross bloodmobile, and he goes home. He has no more nosebleeds.

When Patrick fills out his next MedXPress, he treats the form as if it is a dramatic novel. He exaggerates all his minor issues, including this statement: "ER VISIT: severe nosebleed."

As a result of Patrick's statement, the AME requests his full hospital records, since severe nosebleeds are relatively uncommon and can be associated with other more serious conditions. Patrick gets upset: "But, doc, it was only a little nosebleed!"

The moral of that story is: If you overexaggerate your issues, don't be surprised when medical professionals take your overexaggeration seriously. They can't afford to be wrong. Report things early and report them without adding irrelevant or histrionic details.

▲ ▲ ▲

A gentleman is diagnosed with osteosarcoma and has surgery to remove this cancer. He undergoes treatment and is found to have no evidence of cancer. Astutely, he realizes that even though he is now cured of bone cancer and all his follow-ups have been disease free, he may need some records to give to the FAA.

Thinking the process will be convoluted and onerous, he contacts a company called WeWillSaveYou, Inc., and for a fee of $1,200, he sends them all of his info. These third parties exist under the guise that they will help keep you from losing your medical and guide you through the process. And, yes, they price gouge you, since any good AME would do the same thing for you for a tenth of the cost.

The Third Party sends him a letter in part stating, "This all looks good. Go get your flight physical now; the AME will defer the exam. In about six weeks, we'll contact the FAA and get the FAA reviewers to get you your medical."

As a result, the pilot loses eight weeks of flying, and wastes a lot of money—all the while grumbling about how it was only supposed to take six weeks and believing the sham company when it tells him the FAA is the culprit; sometimes they are *really* slow.

Solution? The moment you are diagnosed with a condition like this, call your AME. The AME will send you a bulleted list of items to send in immediately. You get your treatment, the AME will call the FAA and get verbal authorization to issue you a medical, and you are done.

The take-home message here is simple. Be proactive and involve the decision-maker. Otherwise, you will be disgruntled, and you will complain about the FAA when you yourself were the cause of your own problems. Judgment is a medical problem—the FAA may not have a strict enough yardstick for determining relative amounts of judgment within an individual pilot, but that doesn't make it any less of a medical condition.

There are over twelve hundred accidents in general aviation (GA) per year and over half of them are due to poor judgment. Thus, over seventy-two hundred accidents that have occurred during my period as an AME have been medically related.

Judgment is a medical condition.

5

Math and Myth

or, but I Saw It on the Internet so It Must Be True

RECENT ARTICLES/BLOGS BY vested pilots and their advocates with axes to grind have raised some comical suggestions regarding flight doctors who are against doing away with the third-class medical. These highly inaccurate articles attempt to claim that flight doctors are worried about a loss of income. In fact, that math is never going to work, except where pilots are intentionally going to flight doctors who will pass anything human—alive or inanimate. So what is the math?

Per the FAA's 2014 statistics of pilot medical demographics, there are 351,553 third-class pilots. About 184,000 of those are under age forty and thus need a medical every five years. This equates to about 36,800 exams a year.

Then there are 176,000 over age forty, who need exams every two years. This equates to 88,000 exams a year. Thus, there are approximately 124,800 third-class medicals performed every year.

Now here is the point. There are about three thousand flight doctors. If all things were equal (they aren't), the flight doctors would each do about forty-two third-class flight exams a year.

Obviously, no one is relying upon exams for third-class medicals to create a real business. There are only about twenty doctors in the entire

United States who routinely do over a thousand exams per year (source: AMCD), and these doctors usually do mainly first-class exams, are based in hub cities or near flight schools, and are doing exams on new pilot applicants.

So what is the reality? The reality is that most flight doctors actually have zero financial incentive to keep the third-class medical for two reasons—*economics*, as already discussed, and more importantly, *workload*. The extremely large percentage of pilots over age sixty-five who have multiple, significant diseases (and whom a lot of flight doctors wouldn't even get in the car with to go to the local IHOP), generate a huge net *loss* to the flight doctor in terms of reviewing, reading, lecturing, and teaching.

The net loss is in "time-per-dollar" of revenue generated. There isn't a flight doctor in the world who can't make three times the revenue off a different category of patient than they will off a special-issuance patient over age sixty-five who isn't being forthright or providing information in a timely manner. It isn't difficult to catch the five or six pilots a week lying to you; it is the effort to trying to help them not make a bad situation worse by committing felonies that is extremely time consuming.

Of course, what really happens is that pilots get together and figure out the most easily coerced AME they can find, and they subvert that AME with offers of free flights, dinners, bribes, or other gifts. Then they congregate to this doctor, *knowing* that they have a serious medical issue and *knowing* that as long as the FAA leaves this doctor alone, they will be able to keep flying—and endangering the people they refer to as their loved ones.

So, yes, *those* AMEs that the pilots themselves sought out and built up and who have become protected cronies in a RICO-like conspiracy—those AMEs will have a vested interest and fight against the concept. But they are not a huge number of AMEs.

Loss of income is not the reason most AMEs are against the removal of the third-class medical certification, despite this myth permeating the walls of Congress and the hangars of the local airport. The reason that most AMEs are against the removal of the third-class medical certificate is twofold:

One: They know the DMV isn't qualified currently to certify car licensees.

Two: They have seen more than a few pilots who have severe medical or mental issues, but try to climb into a cockpit with passengers. Anyone who tells you the flight doctor rarely finds anything serious on a flight examination is simply lying or ignorant. There is no other reality. They are either totally dishonest or totally unqualified to make such a statement. Period.

For perspective, I do close to two thousand exams a year and am one of the busiest AMEs in the country. Still, I do only about 190 third-class exams a year and could easily replace that amount of workload with other clientele and be better off financially. Flight exams are only one of my income streams, and my other income streams could easily be ramped up with minimal effort.

But then, I am not an AME who has joined pilots in a conspiracy to defraud the government. The irony is that dishonest pilots create a financial incentive for dishonest AMEs by flocking to them in droves… and then they complain that the persons they enriched are now trying to hold onto their services. Pretty funny stuff.

But, in case, we are misunderstanding the point: the criminal pilot is a subset, not the norm. I'd say 95 percent of pilots are competent, ethical and sane. It is the 5 percent who loudly crash into the schoolhouse or the highway or the building. This is important to remember when reading this book, as it might seem like I am blanketing all pilots under a stereotype with these anecdotes. In fact, the goal is to expose the bad pilots to the light of day, not to paint the good pilots with the same broad brush.

These stories are true anecdotes of actual events, but they only represent a couple of hundred encounters. I have one hundred encounters a week and have been doing this for over seven thousand weeks, so, it is important to understand that there is a subset of pilots that is very dangerous, but there is also a large majority of pilots that is quite competent and ethical.

If most AMEs would simply not complain and let the PBOR2 (Pilot's Bill of Rights 2) pass without clamor, then most AMEs would be a heck of a lot happier after it passes, since then they won't have to deal with patients who act like petulant children while downplaying serious, life-threatening conditions. I know I am going to celebrate the day I can trade my 190 third-class medicals a year for forty Botox patients. They will complain a lot less. (If you don't get that joke, you've never had a lot of Botox patients.)

The true people with a vested interest are twofold: dishonest pilots with poor judgment and flight doctors who have intentionally catered to these pilots and ignored their serious medical issues.

Thankfully, those folks are easy to spot and should be locked up, not rewarded. Interestingly, this is the first time in history that these parties are no longer joined at the hip, as many third-class pilots assert that flight medicals have no value. After all, they claim, pilots have great judgment and should have the right to fly without any real substantive oversight. Meanwhile, a great many of these same pilots demonstrate their great judgment by openly committing felonies every two years by lying on their forms.

Pilot's rights. This is an interesting topic, since at no time in the discussion is an equal right by a hugely outnumbering population mentioned. What about the rights of the landowner? How many people have had their property and their lives destroyed because of the idea that a pilot has a right to fly over their land, when that pilot had no common-sense reason to even be driving a car?

For that matter, how many passengers have been killed by pilots who were flying illegally, impaired, or with pathologically bad judgment?

Well, these are tough statistics to ascertain, but if you extend my study to all GA pilots in the United States, there have probably been well over twelve thousand passengers killed by pilots who shouldn't have been flying on the days that they crashed. (See the chapter on Cessna 172 accidents.)

The federal government is tasked with protecting the general public—with or without the approval of the arrogant eighty-year-old pilot who used to be competent before his advanced Parkinson's/Alzheimer's/seizure/etc., set in, or the arrogant thirty-year-old pilot whose success in business has deluded him into believing that competency translates to all fields. And before you say those people are rare, I will guarantee you, I can walk into any fixed-base operator (FBO) in the country and ask ten people there who the most dangerous pilot on their field is, and six of them will tell me the same name.

I have never once asked a third-class pilot who the most dangerous guy at their airport was without getting an immediate answer. Less regulation isn't the solution to an issue wherein all pilots know we have bad actors who don't belong in the air. The life of the child on the playground that this pilot kills is on every single person at that FBO who knew that pilot was past competency, yet simply talked among themselves like hens in a henhouse and never said a word to the family of the pilot, the feds, etc. It isn't snitching to save people's lives, and it might just save general aviation.

6

Yet More Myths of the Third-Class Medical

or, Trust Me, This Isn't Alzheimer's, My Keys Are in the Goat!

A<small>N EXAMPLE OF</small> a myth, incorrect and not researched as it is, is a recent article by AOPA's flying blog by an editor who has obviously never done one single flight examination. The article declared that *medical reform is finally* coming and the politicians might allow pilots to fly on a document no one on this earth believes is being monitored well enough. Ironically, this article was removed after several months as the writer of the article has moved to a different venue. Perhaps the author's lack of insight into situations regarding aviation extended beyond his clearly wrong insights into medicine.

This gentleman seems to actually believe that flying on a driver's license is a victory. I guess he hasn't heard the term *Pyrrhic victory*. It is actually a political accident (pun intended) waiting to happen, because no one believes the DMV is currently doing a good job, and accident rates are already too high. You don't improve safety by nudging unsafe people into unsafe situations way beyond their competencies. But that is what AOPA is doing…by allowing clueless blog articles like this to be published and by foolishly spreading myths about the third-class medical certification process.

The article, written by a nonphysician who has never performed a single aviation medical examination on a pilot, claimed that, "With rare exceptions…an aviation medical examiner has little or no insight into anything greater than your general health."

This is totally false. Rarely an exam goes by wherein I don't elicit, by careful questioning and by my examination, several issues that a pilot isn't adequately addressing. In fact, it is almost never the case that a pilot over age sixty-five doesn't have two or three hidden gems to uncover with a proper examination. This person's medical training evidently is far different from my own. Now, if you want my opinion of why this AOPA editor thinks the way he does, it is my humble opinion that many pilots, perhaps not him, intentionally seek out AMEs who don't perform careful examinations, and I would say that these pilots look for these characterless doctors because, like birds, they are of the same feather. The very act of intentionally seeking to avoid having an objective medical professional see that you are safe to fly is evidence of a judgment and character issue all by itself. Certainly, you don't take your Cirrus to a shade-tree mechanic.

The article also stated, "One presumes that the purpose of FAA medical standards is to keep pilots who are medically unfit from flying…In some extreme cases they probably do that."

Actually, about five times a week on average, I uncover medically unfit pilot issues, including untreated mental illness, heart disease, obstructed airway, glaucoma, cataracts, etc. On the week I added this sentence, I had five instances.

1. A pilot who lied on his form stating he had no problems at all, and then said to me, "If I wrote down all my problems, I would have to write a book."
2. A pilot who illegally changed the date of his medical.
3. A pilot who brought in records that showed he had had major heart disease for years but had not disclosed it.
4. A pilot who had a mental illness that he hadn't been forthright about previously.
5. Three people who showed up for their flight medicals while ill.

This was a typical week, and all of these items were found during the course of a properly executed medical examination. Such infractions occur weekly, yearly, and year after year.

The AOPA article went on to claim: "But pilots with such conditions almost always ground themselves to begin with." This simply isn't true. I have extensive personal experience with numerous pilots coming to my office after they have been flying with known medical conditions that impair their vision, judgment, coordination, etc. As an objective medical examiner listening to this journalist who has never once treated a pilot medically, my expert medical opinion would be that the writer of the AOPA article was totally wrong about this and was only espousing his biased agenda with a dearth of insight.

Additionally, in reading NTSB reports on every single light-sport fatal accident in the past ten years, it is clear that pilots don't usually ground themselves when they should. In fact, they often kill unwitting and trusting passengers.

The article then states: "Why some drugs were allowed while other drugs with similar profiles and even fewer side effects were banned is a mystery, but it's a mystery that defines the FAA's often arbitrary rules."

This is quite humorous, since the FAA medication decision-making process is not only well thought out and not arbitrary at all, in the one example when they were arbitrary, the decision came back to bite them.

Chantix was promoted as the next big thing in smoking cessation since the *not buying cigerrettes* craze. The FAA jumped on board and waived some of their normal restrictions that they apply to all new medications. Then, Chantix users began having side effects, and the FAA realized it was a bit too arbitrary in bending their own rules. So, the FAA went back to its well thought out strategy of giving a medication shelf time to prove itself and Chantix is no longer allowed because of its occasionally severe side effect profile that could pose a danger to pilots.

And later in the blog came this gem:

"Many pilots with depression were able to get medical clearance from the FAA to fly; it was that a lot of pilots with mild depression were able to stop lying on their application forms."

Us laywriters call this a blatant contradiction.

The AOPA writer explicitly admitted that pilots are routinely dishonest on their exam forms. And he is totally correct, in this one instance.

A subjective depressed pilot's opinion about their level of depression is a fairly silly concept of self-certification. These pilots knew they were taking medication the FAA hadn't approved; they also knew that they had no idea who the FAA hadn't approved these medications. Hell, that was one of the author's other points.

These pilots had no idea whether it was safe to fly on this medication. Some did anyway; others simply didn't take their necessary medication—which meant they more than likely worsened their own depression.

They then lacked all character and morality and lied on a federal application, placing their lives and their passengers' lives at risk, as well as people on the ground, simply because their ignorance and arrogance were affecting their judgment. In fact, this is often the case in depression, wherein people with options are too depressed to recognize their options and commit suicide, often with motor vehicles.

In short, this policy change points out that many pilots absolutely need more oversight because, per the AOPA author, a lot of them are dishonest. All the rules in human history are made because of people like this; hell, you don't need rules for people with character, ethics, and morality—they already know how to behave. You need rules so that you can coerce and then punish the people who refuse to follow any of society's basic premises.

The hilarity of the situation is that their lead general has hoodwinked a lot of other legislators who have not yet figured out that thirty thousand general aviation septuagenarians and their five thousand octogenarian friends are not only a terrible group to hobnob with, when just one mentally ill, formerly competent pilot plows an airplanes into a school or highways you are going to awaken about 330 million people in the United States to your subterfuge, and only about one million give a damn about aviation. Further, no one thinks the DMV is doing a good job with the elderly. Placating an extremely small and highly diseased subset of pilots while endangering the public isn't going to be viewed kindly when reality meets these congressmen.

It would be a political suicide of epic proportions for senators and representatives to not consider that people will well-documented medical conditions take to the skies carrying just a driver's license, intentionally and stupidly endangering the lives of millions. The lies spread by the GA community rabble-rousers about medical examinations not regularly finding important issues are based purely on Goebbelsian propaganda, i.e., total dishonesty without one single shred of truth except for this: the only AMEs that aren't catching medical problems regularly in the elderly third-class pilot group are intentionally doing it and committing crimes, or they simply aren't doing a high volume of elderly pilots.

There is zero truth to the lie that almost all pilots with severe illnesses will self-ground, and even less truth to the lie that light-sport hasn't increased aviation safety hazards. But prove me wrong. Cite one study with the statistical data and research sufficient to lay out your claim. You won't, simply because that study doesn't exist, but the corpses of many LSA passengers and the crumpled carcasses of LSA vehicles certainly do exist, and in a lot larger proportion than their GA cousins.

7

Miscellaneous Anecdotes that Belong Somewhere

or, Doesn't Everyone Else Throw Junk in a Junk Drawer?

D ID YOU KNOW that during the 1800s some guy discovered that water worked better than the medications of the day, so he marketed it and called it *homeopathy*? Well, it's a weird way to say a placebo is better than a bad idea, but there you go.

▲ ▲ ▲

I remember during my internship and residency a urologist who would walk down the corridors. When he saw me at a distance, he'd call out, "Hey, Neil!"

Now, he was a lot of fun to hang out with in surgery and always treated us trainees with respect and honor rather than pretending we were somehow inferior to him, when all we lacked was age, maturity, education, and experience. But, my name isn't Neil; it's John.

This went on for months, but I shrugged it off and didn't really correct him. After all, my name was on my mandatory white coat, my mandatory nametag, and on the surgical daily sheet, etc. Since he was being happy and nice, I wasn't about to rain on his parade.

About a month before I went out into the great big world, he came up, gave me a big hug, and said, "Hey, I know your name is John, John. I just think you look a lot like Neil Diamond." And off he strolled.

And one day, in comes a urology patient, referred to me by my good urologist mentor whom I had a ton of respect for.

"Dr. Shewmaker, my urologist, said to tell Neil hi."

I laughed and said, "Well, next time you see Don Knotts, you tell him hello back for me."

He grinned. "Come to think about it…"

Six weeks later I got a phone call. "You son of a turnip!"—not verbatim—"Neil Diamond was a compliment!"

Now, seriously, I am thinking he was kidding, but…

▲ ▲ ▲

Speaking of the ubiquitous white coat, it has a funny background story. Most people don't realize that it was invented solely for marketing. During the 1800s, people would go to the hospitals where doctors had no real idea about disease, infection, etc. (Read up on Dr. Semmelweis for a good read). Anyway, the white coat was a gimmick that some doctors began using to try to con the public into believing they were better medical professionals as compared to witch doctors, snake oil salesmen, and barbers In fact, until the *Flexner Report* and the advent of the Johns Hopkins's model of modern medical education, death rates simply continued on. Guys in white coats continued killing people with bleeding, huge mixtures of herbal concoctions, and by simply not realizing that speed often trumped sanitation. With the death of diagnosticians and the influx of physician extenders, things appear to be coming back to full circle and rapidly.

In Europe during this period, one doctor's success rate was so high that the other doctors investigated and discovered that he had zero formal training, he was a trained butcher, and his surgical technique was open 'em, fix 'em, close 'em. Meanwhile, the guys in white coats who were killing folks with arrogance and no real cures had finally discovered sanitation, thanks to Semmelweis's suicidal echoes, but they had gone overboard. They would sit with the patient filleted for hours and slowly and carefully operate. And the patient would die of infection from being exposed for too long.

My favorite personal white-coat story happened when I was sitting in a lecture hall, listening to an expert in child psychology. He was an excellent speaker, but kinda ruined it from the start. "You medical students are sitting here in scrubs and street clothes and flip-flops, and that isn't very professional," he said, and he dragged on this line of thought for a few minutes until he evidently realized that a nonsurgical psychiatrist wearing scrubs was sort of antithetical to the points he was trying to make, and he uttered a line too rich not to pass on. "Now, I am here today in scrubs, but I have earned that right. I have undergone years of education, residency, and training."

My hand shot up. "At what point in one's career does one earn the right to dress unprofessionally?"

I really don't think he liked that question, but it did shift him into focusing more on the very good lecture he then gave on how to spot abuse. I still wonder if we need to have a scrubs ceremony for when our training and expertise has reached a level of such acumen that we have earned the right not to the dress the way we believed it was paramount that we dress the day before. The National Institutes of Health (NIH) needs to study this…right after it gets those shrimp off the treadmills.

▲ ▲ ▲

One day a pilot came to my office. As we were preparing him for his ECG, he let me know that he ran marathons and he had been in the navy.

"Doc, my heart rate is in the forties, and every time I'd get a navy exam, my ECG would be too slow. Then they'd make me do jumping jacks, and at that point, I'd begin having extra heartbeats, and then they'd send me off to have other tests."

So I thought, *Gee, thanks. Now I am nervous*, but I hooked him up to the machine. Turns out, he was at forty-nine beats per minute, and the FAA standard for heart rates at that time was fifty. Internally, I thought, *Aww…crud,* but then I had a moment of inspiration.

I leaned down and whispered, "Tell me about your ex-wife." His heart rate went up to fifty; I pressed the button and got a perfect ECG.

We'll ignore the topic of the federal government doing massive, unnecessary ECG testing on young men. (I mean the navy; the FAA concept, while still overkill, is at least based on a model that once existed and had a period of being in vogue...forty years ago.)

▲ ▲ ▲

Another time on an ECG, I pressed the run button and got the following prompt: "arm leads reversed." I didn't bother to look; I just took the left lead and moved it to the right arm and vice versa. Still, "arm leads reversed." So I, being astute and professional, began grumbling, mumbling, and harrumphing...all with an impressive expression of confusion. I did two or three more switches, but the patient simply wasn't made for that particular machine. The heart was OK, but the electronics and the software just didn't match the patient.

▲ ▲ ▲

Another time, I put the purple lead where the blue lead was supposed to go, perhaps not having the best lighting on the chest wall. The machine read that the patient was having a heart attack. Luckily I was able to figure out, after a bit of head scratching, that I was giving the guy a heart attack—both by wiring him wrong and then scaring him into a heart attack because of it. Over time and repetition, you learn: if it reads abnormal, slow down and recheck all the leads before you start a process that can be both unneeded and expensive.

Anecdotally, I do hear from lots of pilots that other AMEs will simply just do the first ECG and if it is abnormal, well, too bad. Hopefully, those anecdotes aren't true, because that would be a real stain on my profession.

▲ ▲ ▲

Color-blindness is a source of occasional anecdotes. Many AMEs are accused by pilots of cheating and simply pointing out colors on the wall. Is this true? Who knows, but many pilots (maybe four or five a year) will call up and ask if we have a Farnsworth lantern, because that is the only test they can pass. It always comes out that their AME doesn't have a Farnsworth, but they at one time told that AME that they had passed the Farnsworth, and thus the AME took this as gospel.

When I explain the very simple way they can get a color-blind waiver, many simply hang up, upset with me. The truth is, they have usually gamed the system so long that now they are afraid to come out and have the issue fixed. A blanket, free color-vision waiver day at all the local Flight Standard District Offices (FSDOs) to grandfather-in this fairly large minority of pilots (I'd guess it's about two or three thousand) might just put that issue to bed.

More often, the pilot will show up and immediately state that they have a lot of trouble with the color charts. No warning, just act like my best friend all the way up to, "Doc, I can't really do these colors, can you just point some out."

Yeah, and not even an envelope of cash to go along with the coercion.

What most pilots need in this case is a simple: a calm explanation that most of the time, their past examiners simply have failed them too soon. The fields on the color-vison tests are three dimensional, and if you ask them to focus carefully for a minute or two without actually trying to give an answer and then answer, they will often do just fine.

▲ ▲ ▲

The best incident was the seventy-year-old ex-FAA employee who had been waivered for being color-blind for forty-plus years. He sat in the eye machine (not because he had to, but because we were both curious) and he just sat there. No word would come out of his mouth. Nothing. And no amount of prodding would do it. I looked at his form, and it stated "retired engineer." I had a sudden moment of rare clarity.

I pretended my finger was a gun, put it to his head, and said, "Look, you are in a hostage situation. I will shoot if you don't answer something, so tell me immediately the numbers that you think are there." He got every single number right and quickly.

The insight that I had is that he was an engineer, and like land surveyors, engineers tend to be extremely resistant to giving wrong answers. He took this to the next level by refusing for forty years to ever answer an eye-chart question unless he was absolutely sure. This is, of course, the opposite of how a bunch of variable circles of different colors is supposed to be read. It basically begs you to make an educated guess. He was too educated to fall for that. Once I made him answer, he was magically cured of his color blindness.

▲ ▲ ▲

Sometimes the anecdotes occur when you send a pilot to get reports. This can be quite fun, since many specialists don't mind getting paid for an hour-long surgery, but ask them to write a two-paragraph status report that is spelled out in detail, and they act as if you are giving them new math on their first day of middle school. This is despite the fact that they have zero problems writing three-page consultation reports when their reimbursement is guaranteed. It is pretty sad at times to watch. I can only imagine the reports AMCD (aerospace medical certification division) and the regional flight surgeons receive regularly.

One day, I sent a pilot to get a status report and it came back on blank paper—no date, no letterhead. The status report was about two hundred words. Pretty good, right? Except it was smudged because it was in pencil. From the VA. I kid you not. Of course, if you have ever wasted your time while the VA doc puts into the computer all the answers to whether there are guns in your home, how many dogs you eat, or if you have any domestic violence issues (after noting you're single), then you know it isn't like they don't have the resources to put a one-paragraph status report on a letterhead.

A lot of times, a physician will get lazy and simply write: "patient's thyroid well controlled, TSH normal," and then (this happens three or four times a year) you ask for the labs that weren't included and find the TSH isn't normal at all. Of course, this could be coercion by the pilot upon the physician or their staff, but the bottom line is, it happens way too much.

When the CACI (Conditions under which AME Can Issue) protocols came out, I routinely would print off my checklist and give it to a pilot, and three or four times, the doc would just write "OK," or "agreed" and sign their name to that. I had to start telling pilots I wouldn't accept the paper that way, so do not let the doctor simply write "OK" or "Bob is fine" on it. Brevity is good, but laziness is its evil twin.

In fact, this must happen a lot, as I remember one FAA directive specifically reminding all of us AMEs that "Bob is OK" isn't a good enough status report.

In an effort to template the requests so as not to confuse these post-graduate, highly trained physicians who routinely write long consultations, I at one time, would write a sample letter. I had to make sure I didn't use the pilot's name or the doctor's name or these would come back marked "agreed" and that would be their idea of a status report.

8

Beyond Judgment

or, I Don't Think They Planned to Be Sociopaths, but That's Where the Path Led

Some events just go so far beyond poor judgment that they deserve a chapter and/or a straitjacket of their own.

One Saturday morning, my son and I arrived to do a batch of student pilot physicals. There were about eight pilots scheduled, so we knew we were going to be there all morning. They were scheduled to arrive at 9:00 a.m. This had all been preplanned with the flight school.

As the clock ticked past the hour, my son and I grew more and more upset. To add to the situation, the flight school didn't answer the phone. We also had a pilot coming in at noon, so we decided to surf the web while we waited. Around ten thirty, the school bus arrived with its eight pilots and a very young driver.

I was a bit irate about this obvious rudeness—not calling, dragging us to the office an hour and half early on the weekend, and leaving us with no idea if they are even coming. I asked the driver why he hadn't called.

"Well, they only told me to pick them up at eight thirty to take them to the doctor. They didn't tell me when they had to arrive, so I took them to Walmart and breakfast."

At that point, I was thinking there wasn't much hope for this kid, but perhaps I was pessimistic. But when I explained to him that we weren't on this earth for him to trample us, he responded with, "I don't like your attitude. Let's go—"

And he then attempted to take the pilots back to the flight school. At that point, I explained he could just as easily have been a horse and buggy or an automated zip line, and his role was over the moment the pilots left the van.

He was welcome to wait outside for them, but he wasn't about to become important in the decision-making process about their exams and who would be doing them. So out of the office he went, and into the office came the poor, confused students who'd thought they were getting medicals but instead had waited in Walmart while their driver texted all morning and ate a breakfast muffin. I never did find out what the reaction of the flight school management was when he tried to explain why he'd picked up the students but did not deliver them promptly, when that was the only role they'd given him when they allowed him to use their company vehicle.

▲ ▲ ▲

One day, the lobby was full of patients, and a guy walked up after parking his semitruck. He promptly threw a cigarette under my car and opened the door to my office.

I said, "Jesus Christ! How much do you smoke?" (because there is nothing fouler than a smoker walking into a small office), and he looked all confused.

"Uh, do you mean cigarettes?"

So now the entire lobby was laughing and I acted serious and said, "No, I mean pot!" I was, of course, expecting a denial, since clearly I was joking.

But he said, "Oh, pot? About a joint or two a week. I smoke about a pack a day of cigarettes."

Yeah, I'm thinking I may have to review HIPAA after that one. Sometimes you have to pick your spots.

▲ ▲ ▲

Some things happen before you even get into your car to go to work. One day, I walked out to get into my car, and a lady was letting her dog urinate on my trashcan.

"What the—do the freaking trees around here only take reservations?"

She failed her pilot physical just by walking her dog in front of my house…I am still waiting for her to show up at the office so I can fail her. I wonder if she knows about the online schedule…

▲ ▲ ▲

On another day, the state of Florida's new rules ran afoul of a dying truck driver. About two years ago, the FDOT made a rule change, stating that drivers who have a trucking endorsement on their licenses must maintain a DOT medical. Well, that swelled my practice, as lots of licensed drivers who weren't actively using their commercial endorsements suddenly had to rush to get a medical—not because they wanted to use their endorsement, but just because they wanted to keep the endorsement in case they might need it in the future. Now, obviously, this is a ridiculous and unneeded rule by FDOT, but nonetheless, I did a lot of new DOT physicals.

The extent to which a person wishes to maintain an endorsement has its limit in common sense, however. One gentleman came in with no voice at all because he had just been diagnosed with throat cancer and had started chemotherapy. He kept falling asleep in my lobby because he was totally exhausted, but he didn't want to lose that endorsement. He wasn't going to use it, he really didn't need a medical for it because if he did drive commercially and didn't have an active medical, the punishment for that crime was already in place.

▲ ▲ ▲

The strangest one I remember was when a gentleman walked in, filled out his forms, and stated he was on antidepressants, antiseizure meds, narcotics, etc. He was a very honest and open young man, about twenty-nine years old. I asked him about his disclosures, and he stated that he had Glioblastoma Multiforme, had had debulking brain surgery, and experienced weekly seizures.

He had a commercial endorsement, however, and didn't want to lose it, so here he was for a DOT medical, even though legally he wasn't able to drive a moped on the road. To this day, I don't think he understood why I couldn't help him, although I felt for him, having lost my mother to Glioblastoma and having studied this terrible disease incessantly for months as part of my way of dealing with my own personal sense of helplessness.

Hopefully, in moments of clarity when he isn't fully dosed on narcotics as he was that day, I have a selfish wish that he understands I wasn't being villainous but was simply trying to protect him from his own illusions.

▲ ▲ ▲

One day a gentleman that I had never spoken with or seen called me. "John," he asked, "if I send my information to AMCD, will I get an answer about my heart surgery back within five weeks?"

"Well, when does your medical expire?"

"Oh, it's been expired for several months. I had heart surgery, and I've been waiting six months to fly again."

Oh, good. He gets the concept, I thought. "Well, sir, it may take six weeks, or maybe eight; it really isn't easy to guess."

"Oh, to hell with this," he groused. "I am just going to go fly my airplane anyway."

Thunk, thunk, thunk.

"Well, that's great sir. Good luck committing a federal crime after admitting on a phone line to a gentleman you have never met that you intend to commit a felony."

Click…bzzz.

▲ ▲ ▲

A pilot's wife called up one day: "Why can't my husband fly if his HA1C is over nine? He wants to get his flight medical, but his HA1C is about 9.6."

"Well, ma'am, it means he is at a highly elevated risk for diabetic complications, a much higher risk of heart attack, and so on."

"Well, that's not true. I am a nurse, and that's just not true."

"Where are you a nurse, hospice?" (That was an afterthought, clearly I am not that quick.)

▲ ▲ ▲

Another day, a young lady called up to ask about flight exams. "Hey, my boyfriend wanted me to ask, what does the FAA think if a person does acid?"

I replied, "They probably won't see things the same way he would."

▲ ▲ ▲

Another day I was giving an overweight pilot an ECG. I was talking to him about weight loss, when he said, "Oh, I don't care if I die or live; if it's going to happen, it's going to happen."

ECG turns out abnormal.

"Oh my God! Does this mean I am going to die?" And he began a complete reversal of the "who cares; life happens" attitude.

Turns out it was just a variant he'd always had. Two years later, he still hadn't lost weight. He came in and told me he went to have a stress test, but then he refused to tell me why.

I asked for records, and he refused. He said, "I knew this was going to be that way, and you are just looking for an excuse to fail me," and stormed out.

Hmm, wonder what that was all about.

▲ ▲ ▲

Another guy failed to bring any of his medical info for about the eighth straight time, even though he was on a special issuance. I had repeatedly educated him carefully with bulleted lists about what he needs to send and that he needs to do this well in advance of his exam, to no avail. I send him off again to get all the stuff, and he stormed out.

"You always make me drive here several times," he complained.

I replied, "Well, like I told you the last seven times, if you want to e-mail this stuff to me well in advance of your exam, I could take a look and let you know if it is all there."

"You've never told me that!"

Hmm…let's see. "Well, maybe you're correct…No, actually I have about a dozen well-written e-mails in my SENT file that you have responded to in the past."

What does he say next? "You are just looking for reasons to fail me!"

*Hmm…*made me wonder a little. Yeah, buddy, that is a wonderful business plan. Intentionally failing pilots who could pass if they'd simply follow basic directions isn't a great retirement plan for flight doctors.

A week later, a nasty online review about how I was just trying to fail pilots appeared on the Internet. Ironically my practice grew that year by about three hundred pilots, mostly by word of mouth and targeted advertising, and the practice continued to grow for eight more years. The squeaky wheel was ignored.

▲ ▲ ▲

Then there's this guy. He spent fifteen minutes trying to find *United States* on the drop-down box for citizenship. I told him it's there; it starts with a *U*. It's *USA*.

"Oh! It's abbreviated," he cried.

I was telling this story once, and another pilot said, "Makes you wonder what he yells at the Olympics, doesn't it?"

▲ ▲ ▲

A lot of times (and I mean a lot of times!), pilots will come in from out of town and have medical issues, medication issues, new problems, and so on, without bringing any paperwork, yet they will pressure you to pass them.

One day, a guy walked in for an appointment and stated to me that he hasn't flown in a long time but is on metformin for diabetes.

He said, "I want a first-class medical because I have a job offer at a training facility."

I told him he needs forms A, B, C, D, and E.

"But why?" he protests. "I didn't need those the last time."

"When were you diagnosed with diabetes?" I ask.

"Six years ago."

"And when did you have your last medical?"

"Twelve years ago." There was a pause, and then he said, "Sir, your lower lip is bleeding."

"I am biting it," I said. "It's a bad habit I seem to do far too often." Anyway, it gets better.

The pilot asked me to talk directly to his doctor, so I did and told them what to fax over.

Two days later, I got a fax from his doctor out in the badlands of the west, and the son of a gun is on insulin. So I called the pilot who was staying on the other side of town to ask him about this. I had spent over an hour explaining to him the different variants of medications for diabetes and how that would affect him getting his medical. I'd told him that noninsulin-dependent diabetics (such as he) needed A, B, C, and D, and handed him a form for pilots with noninsulin dependent diabetes, so he could understand the FAA regulations regarding persons with that condition.

"Insulin," he said. "I didn't know that was for diabetes. I thought that was for my blood pressure, and I forgot to put that on the list!"

"If you see a spurt of blood on the horizon, don't pay it too much attention. I am really biting my lip at the moment." Just a thought, of course.

I call folks like him and the "oh, it's abbreviated" guy my Six Sigma applicants, because I am almost 100 percent certain that 99.9 percent of all flight doctors have never had a patient with a six-year history of diabetes on insulin with numerous visits to the doctor and the pharmacy try to tell the AME, "Oh, I thought that thing I was daily injecting was for my freaking blood pressure!"

But if you are going to get caught in a lie, I guess you go big or stay home. The "oh, it's abbreviated!" guy is a lot less of a medical risk, of course.

▲ ▲ ▲

Some bad judgments happen a lot, like those pilots who know they have a problem but still come to the exam. Probably six to seven times a year, I find a new discovery—cataracts. But about five of those times, the pilots admit they knew something was wrong with that eye…or both of them.

▲ ▲ ▲

Some funny things regarding possible mental issues happen outside of the office.

One night I was giving a talk at an EAA meeting, when a guy raised his hand and asked in the open forum, "Hey, when is the FAA going to quit making people stop flying just because they drink?"

"Why?" I responded.

"Well, they say I am an alcoholic, but I don't agree at all."

This is in an open room with a ton of people, so I thought, *Sir, you may not be an alcoholic, but your judgment of when to ask a question may be a bit skewed.*

▲ ▲ ▲

Another day, I was looking at a seventy-year-old man's freshly healed umbilical scar (blind stab). "Why are you trying to hide your prostate surgery?" I asked.

"Oh, man," he cried. "How did you know about that?"

"Well, the recent surgical scars around your umbilicus for one, and two, you told me."

▲ ▲ ▲

Another gentleman spent the entire exam with his pants around his lower ribs. I made him lower them, and there was the colostomy bag.

It makes me wonder if AOPA writers really care about how often pilots lie on their exams. Based on their lack of research and blatantly wrong comments, I am guessing that wouldn't meld well with their agenda.

▲ ▲ ▲

Another day, a guy called me on the phone fifteen minutes after the exam. "Hey," he said, "what would happen if someone had a heart attack and didn't disclose it?"

"Well, I am not sure," I replied. "I'll ask the FAA for you and have them call you back with the answer."

Sometimes, people want to tell the truth. It just takes a little coaxing. That is often the humor of it—they *want* to tell you, but they want you to understand why they have been lying, so it becomes comedic in how they then rationalize. And let me tell you, when it comes to rationalizing, no one is better at it than the obese pilot. But then, no one is better at not buying a bag of cow dung than an AME who knows that rationalization doesn't equal reality. Thus, we will gorge ourselves on the topic of obesity on another day.

9

And *You* Want to Fly *My* Airplane?

or, Is It Easier to Go to New York or by Train?

Sometimes, you seriously have to question whether a person should be flying airplanes.

 Me: When did you have the brain surgery?
 Pilot: Oh, about the time we lived in Oklahoma.
 Me: Was that before or after Aunt Mildred fell off the horse?
 Pilot: Who is Aunt Mildred?
 Me: The only person in my whole family who knows when you were ever in Oklahoma.

What very common object weighs more on the moon than on the earth? A balloon.

▲ ▲ ▲

Another day, an English gentleman walked in and I asked him for a picture ID.

"What do you mean," he asked.

"You know, your passport, a driver's license. A picture ID."

He said, "I'll be back…"

An hour later, he came back and plopped two passport photos he just had made at the CVS pharmacy onto my desk

"You said you needed a photo," he said to my blank stare.

And that is when I knew a second-story office had a drawback. There will be times when you are tempted to jump out the window just so you can laugh out loud.

▲ ▲ ▲

Guy: I am at 5214. There is a 5212, but no 5213.
Me: Uh, sir…it's across the street.

Another time:

Guy: I'm at 5568 Hoffner. Are you guys east or west?
Me: Sir, walk to the next building…OK, what's the number?
Guy: 5560.
Me: Good. We're that way; keep coming…but drive really slow.

And another time:

Guy: Hey, I am on Semoran [Conway] [I-95]. Do I turn left or right onto your road?
Me: Sir, are you going south or north?

And again:

Guy: Hey, I am at 404, and there is a 406. No 405.
Me: Other side of the building.

▲ ▲ ▲

I watched a guy push on my door. He stood back, looked at my office for five minutes, then called. "Is your office open?"

"Yeah, pull on the door."

▲ ▲ ▲

Lady called at 6:17 p.m.: "I am outside of your office, and it is closed."
"Yes, ma'am. We are closed."
"But I had a six o'clock appointment."
"Yes. We left at ten minutes after."
"Wow!" *Click.*

▲ ▲ ▲

A common phone call starts with, "You spelled my name wrong on my medical!"

"Uh, sir, you typed your name into the system." It happens a lot actually, we are all human.

Actually, the funny one is when young, male, Spanish-speaking pilots are filling out the online form. They often will put *Sr.* after their name in the computer because they think it means *señor,* so I make sure to ask them about their children, and we get it all straightened out.

▲ ▲ ▲

Pilot tried repeatedly to grab the mail flap to open the door. He bumped his head on the door.

*Hmm...*yep, smelled a bit like he'd been drinking.

▲ ▲ ▲

Here was a guy complaining about the good old days, so I asked him to give an example.

"Well," he said, "I was walking down the Jetway at MCO, and this lady was there with her son. He tugged on her skirt and said, 'Look, Mom, it's the pilot!' I said, 'Excuse me, I am the captain.'"

I paused for a second's worth of thought, but I really wanted to roll on the floor. I bit my tongue, made my tone soft, almost flat and emotionless. OK, here went me:

"Oh, that sounds devastating." *Whirr.* The comment flew right over his head.

▲ ▲ ▲

Guy complained that you can't call 'em *stews* and that the good-looking young'uns are all guys.

Me: You didn't get the memo?
Pilot: Huh?
Me: Sleeping with them isn't mandatory to your job requirements.

Whirr...right over his head. There is value in keeping a straight face.

▲ ▲ ▲

Every month I will get a call from a desperate pilot. "Would you be able to drive to your other office today?" It's two hours away.

A couple of times a year, we'll hear on a Sunday, "Could you come in today?"

▲ ▲ ▲

Sometimes, even a well-placed, well-explained sign telling pilots not to leave the bathroom with their urine isn't foolproof.

I was standing in the hallway, drinking a large diet Coke. Pilot walked out of the bathroom and right up to me with his urine cup.

Me: Get back into the bathroom.
Pilot: Your sign confused me.
Me: Read it out loud; I am out here listening.
Pilot: You are standing in a bathroom. Urine belongs in a bathroom. Put the cup of urine down and flush the toilet. Wash hands and leave the cup in the bathroom.

Me: So, why do you think a sign needs to be in the bathroom in the first place?
Pilot: What, did people use to carry it out or something?
Me: Yep, right up to me when I am trying to drink a soda, even.

Four times that has happened since the sign went up. Most of the time, the pilots read the sign, and you can tell because you hear them chuckle. Sometimes they don't read the sign.

On four occasions, pilots have read the sign that tells them to leave the urine in the bathroom, and the sign confused them.

▲ ▲ ▲

One Saturday, I put on my adult clothing and stumbled off to a loss-leader exam. By eleven o'clock, he hadn't shown up. I figured I'd wait fifteen minutes more and out I'd go.

Phone rang at 11:10 a.m. "Doc, I'm not going to make it, the plane is broken down…up here…in New York."

My office is in Florida, so this guy had known for the past three hours he wouldn't be at my office at eleven o'clock.

▲ ▲ ▲

Or another time, a guy called me at 6:23 p.m. "Hey, I had a six o'clock appointment, and you guys have the door locked."

"Yes, sir, we leave after five minutes if the last person hasn't bothered to call."

"Five minutes! But I was only twenty minutes late!"

God forbid we leave our office ever when someone is late but doesn't call. Of course we will stay there until sunrise for that person.

▲ ▲ ▲

I looked in a guy's ear. "How much do you smoke?"
"A pack a day. How did you know?"
"You just told me."

▲ ▲ ▲

Guy was holding his arms above his head…well, one of them, at least.
"When'd you hurt your arm?"
"Since childhood. Wow, you are good!"
"Uh, sir, you can't raise your arm over your head, and I am good at figuring that out?"

He was a very accomplished pilot, but the injury wasn't documented. That could have been a potential issue for the pilot later. So we got him all righteous with a quick call to FAA.

Most times when a gentleman can't lift an arm, it is because of an ongoing injury that they're trying to cover up. This happens quite a bit, and when these mostly third-class pilots get called on it, they usually admit they were planning on fixing it or maybe having it evaluated sometime. They also admit that they've flown repeatedly and that it was a lot harder to do than normal. Yeah, AOPA certainly wouldn't know about this very frequent kind of pilot decision-making would they?

▲ ▲ ▲

Guy lying on ECG table asked, "So, are you in this office today?"
"Read the bottom line of the eye chart, please."
"You mean the very bottom one?"
"Yep." So the pilot did it, and I asked, "OK, now read the other bottom line you were talking about before."

▲ ▲ ▲

Patient handed me a form showing she used levothyroxine. I asked, "How long have you been diagnosed with hypothyroidism?"

"Wow," she said. "You are good."

▲ ▲ ▲

Guy standing in front of the office asked, "Is the office open today?"

"Yes."

"OK. I'll make an appointment online then and come back."

▲ ▲ ▲

Guy standing in front of the office called me on my phone. "Is the office open today?"

"Yes."

"Well, the door's closed."

"Sir, it is seven forty in the morning. You woke me up!"

▲ ▲ ▲

"I ish here fur mah flighhhying esham..."

There are actually pilots who drink alcohol at lunch and then come in for their flight exams. Some will hang out until three with their friends and then come in. This has slowed a lot in recent years, so either judgment is improving, punishment is improving, or word of mouth is keeping all the drinkers away from my office.

▲ ▲ ▲

Sometimes silly things happen, and I realize I am all alone. Like, I am playing in the stock market so sending the money all out to my brokerage house...and then realize I haven't paid the cable bill and my TV is cut off on the first day of football season…and God forbid I use one of my seven or eight credit cards…*hmm*. This is uncomfortable. Let's stick to other people and the things they do; no one wants to hear about the time I drove someone to a car place to drop off their car…in the car we were planning to drop off.

▲ ▲ ▲

Guy wanted me to backdate his medical form. He had an out-of-date medical and was out on bail. He told officials he'd lost it. I'd never seen the guy in my life, but he was arrested at 2:00 a.m. on a darkened airstrip, because he was found with an airplane with a strong smell of pot and some seeds in the floorboards.

▲ ▲ ▲

Pilot walked into the bathroom. Instead of picking up a cup from the pile of cups to pee in, he opened the urine testing strip bottle and pees on my brand-new strips, filling the strip bottle. It would have been far worse if it were a narrow-mouthed bottle.

▲ ▲ ▲

I told a pilot I needed two drops of urine…and son of a gun, if he didn't spend fifteen minutes and come out with exactly two drops of urine. I use a TB syringe and tested him—one drop on glucose, one drop on protein.

▲ ▲ ▲

Pilot rushed into the bathroom on his thirtieth visit to me. "Gotta go, doc!" He didn't use the cups and had to wait two hours to get his sample.

▲ ▲ ▲

Pilot showed up, and his wife was within half a foot of him the entire visit; she even wanted to go into the very small bathroom with him. That's where I draw the line. A Siamese twin by choice not design is a medical red flag. Not sure where it's going to lead, but it's going to cause a journey of exploration to begin. Bet on it.

▲ ▲ ▲

Pilot showed up with his urine already in a cup. "But I'm shy, doc," he said.

His wife who was with him nodded. "Yeah, doc, he's shy."

I suddenly looked to see if anyone standing next to me had on an I'M NEXT TO STUPID shirt.

▲ ▲ ▲

Pilot showed up in a shoulder sling with a broken clavicle. "I'm here to get my flight medical," he said. Not so much.

▲ ▲ ▲

Pilot showed up; I asked him for MedXPress number. His wife was standing very close. He turned and had her get her phone out of her purse and read it to me. I put the confirmation number in the system. He hadn't flown for seven years.

"Yep, looking for new opportunity," he said.

"Where are you from?"

"Oh, the Carib, you know, the island—" He names one of the many non-US islands.

"OK, so do you have a picture ID?"

"What do I need a picture ID for?"

"It's a federal exam. It's required."

"But I didn't bring it."

"No license? No passport?"

The pilot then started getting really mad at me. Inside I was laughing, because he was also telling me something else was going on here. Why?

Well, the wife never sat down. She hovered next to him, she was handling his business, and he had no ID. He was a foreigner with no ID, and he was getting mad at me because he doesn't have ID for a government medical exam in a country he isn't a part of?

So, this isn't rocket science. He was either a total mental case or there was more to the story…and he left all mad. I got curious—which is never good—and looked up his name on Google Images. Surprise! He had a picture ID the whole time…his mug shot.

▲ ▲ ▲

Guy came in with another guy (that happens occasionally), but this guy had been to see me several times and had never done this before. He said the other guy has to drive him because he had an altercation with a cop. I asked if it was drugs or alcohol.

"Nope, not at all," he assured me. Routine stop; he and the cop had words, they confiscated his license, booked him for being disorderly, and he had to go to court the next week. But not anything to do with drugs or alcohol…nope.

As it turned out, it was not just alcohol. It was his third arrest, and the guy tried to tell the FAA that *I* had told him that this wasn't a big deal and he didn't have to do anything about it.

That came back to haunt him in a big way, and I got to have fun laughing with a nice FAA attorney who couldn't believe I could remember the details from a year prior, but I knew the pilot and I remembered that he usually didn't come in with anyone, yet that time he did. That memory stuck like gum.

▲ ▲ ▲

Pilots love rumors and myths: the sleep apnea myths are hilarious, skinny guys with big necks even get all flustered and bothered, just myths spreading like a fungus. Myths are ubiquitous to aviation.

"Why won't the FAA let you fly on blood pressure meds?" One pilot asked in the middle of a safety seminar, and immediately the rest of the room started talking. See, the FAA lets you fly with controlled hypertension, and half of them were taking blood pressure medication. I think the gentleman had listened to a hangar expert and never asked an AME.

A pilot walked into the office and left parts of the form blank. I asked why, and he said, "I want to keep those things private."

Another pilot walked into the office and left "hospital and other illness" blank. I asked why.

"Do they want all of my injuries?" he asked incredulously.

"Yes, sir, they do."

"But I rode motocross..."

Yep, I could see his point.

▲ ▲ ▲

Best one liners:

"OK sir, I am going to see if you remember my three rules. You should never ask me to do anything..."

Pilot one: Period!
Pilot two: Ever!
Pilot three: Free?

▲ ▲ ▲

Patient: My *real* doctor thinks...
Ouch!

Patient: What is your specialty?
Me: Evasion.

▲ ▲ ▲

Another guy insisted that his AOPA doctor said that I could do his hypertension report. "I don't know you, sir. So no, I can't."

▲ ▲ ▲

One day I was reading an ECG strip: bradycardia (and seeing his heart rate was at 54).

Me: Sir, you have a normal ECG, but due to your exercising, you probably have always had a slow heart rate.
Guy: But I was told in the past it was abnormal. They said it was… b-, um…something that started with a B.
Me: Yes, sir, you do have bradycardia.
Guy: Yeah, that's it. But no one's ever told me what it means.
Me: It's Latin for you have a slow heart rate, sir.
Guy: Oh, sheesh! Why didn't they say that? I always have that. I run marathons!

▲ ▲ ▲

A different day, reading an ECG:

Me: You have a right bundle branch block.
Patient: You are really good.

▲ ▲ ▲

Recently, a gentleman was looking into the near-vision machine to test his vision.

Patient: Can you focus that for me?
Me: Uh, sir, it is an eye test to see if *your eyes* can focus.

▲ ▲ ▲

Sometimes the best communication is to hang up the phone. There are days when I might call and ask, "Who is on duty at AMCD?" When the FAA subcontractor tells me it's Dr. X, I hang up the phone and move on.

(I mean no offense to the FAA folks reading this; it's just some things require a hammer and some a feather pillow.)

Certain things, you want certain doctors for. Most cases it won't matter; the facts and the records are what they are. But every once in a while, you see a small problem in front of you and a big problem on paper, and you want someone who will listen to your point of view—not drown out your thoughts.

If there is one thing you might learn from reading this, it's that doctors can have egos, especially ones that ruffle when questioned. If I have all my ducks lined up, then I know almost to a word the exact questions the person on the other end is going to ask. If they let me lay it out and if I've done my legwork, we will have a fast phone call. But if their day is slow and mine isn't...all I can say is, thank God the phones aren't all video phones, because the faces I am making while they are talking sometimes aren't appreciated beyond my cranium.

▲ ▲ ▲

Sometimes, school physicals can give you a good belly laugh.

I once asked a young man to read the bottom line of the eyechart, which is the following: P-E-Z-O-L-C-F-T-D

The young man sounded out, "Pezulfud?"

Well, that was a pretty good attempt at reading the eye chart. He didn't know the meaning of the word *pezulfud* though, so we went back and tried it one letter at a time.

10

First-Time Problems

or, Why You Shouldn't Pretend Your Flight Doctor Is as Dumb as You've Heard

ONE DAY A seventy-seven year old gentleman walked in and sat down. I said, "So, I see your last medical was twenty years ago. What gets you interested in flying again?"

"Well, my son is buying an airplane and—"

"When is the last time you went to a doctor?"

"Oh, I never go to the doctor; they only try to find things wrong with you. I hate doctors." (Time to use a twenty-first centuryism…"SMH!")

So I said, "Well, let's see what we can do…" I began listening to his heart, and I heard a consistently irregular beat—almost like the heart beat twice, paused, and then did it again. This can be a few things—it can be caused by several heart issues, but I've seen it in heavy coffee drinkers a couple of times, too. So I told him (because I am a smart guy and not shy about proving it), "OK, listen to my heart." I let him listen. Then I moved the stethoscope to his chest. "Now, listen to your heart." He did. "Which one sounds strange to you?"

"You found something wrong! I knew it!"

So I said, "But did *you* hear any difference?"

"Yeah," he said. "What's going on with my heart?"

"I don't know. You are the one who thinks there may be a problem. I haven't said a word about it having a problem. All I did was ask you to listen to our hearts. I do have an ECG machine, though, and it has a computer in it that tells us info. Let's see if *it* thinks you're right. We need to find out if you are right about you having a problem in your heart, so let's see if this machine can tell us anything."

By now he was fuming because he couldn't accuse me of diagnosing him with a heart issue, because *he* said his heart sounds unusual, not me.

Yeah, tricky, but…it is what it is, right?

So we hooked him up and find he had couplets. By itself, this didn't prove anything, but in the setting of a seventy-seven-year-old who hated doctors and likely wouldn't be that prone to openly admitting any known issues—this was a situation that required finesse.

But I was the only one there, so I dove right in.

"Sir, I don't know what exactly is causing your arrhythmia, but you need to have a full cardiology work-up. The good news is that this isn't atrial fibrillation." (I had pretty much known that because of the regularity of the irregularity, but I needed to give him some good news to go with the bad, and most older people who watch TV hear about atrial fibrillation without really knowing what it is, so it got to be my bogeyman.)

He got his feathers fluffed, and his chest started turning red. He looked like a male prairie grouse about to attract a female, and this scared me…well, at least I found it unattractive. I said, "Look, let's take a bigger view of this. Yes, this is a new thing you have found when you listened to your heart, but if this is a serious heart issue, you may have just added twenty years to your life by you catching it."

"Well, then I'll come back in twenty f-ing years and say thank you then!"

The good news is, the guy's wife sent me a card five weeks later, thanking me and informing me his triple bypass went well. He also came back in six months, got his medical with a special issuance, and two subsequent ones into his early eighties, until we lost touch. I have about thirteen years still to wait to see if he carries through on returning to thank me, but I hope he can make it. Hell, at least he didn't land on a runway marked X with men and equipment on it.

▲ ▲ ▲

Sometimes, the flight doctor does such an impressive job that the pilot will begin referring other pilots. This can be a double-edged sword, because while pilot referrals are very much appreciated, that is dependent upon the new pilot possessing great judgment...or marginal judgment...maybe some judgment, at the very least? However, that isn't always the case, as illustrated in my next story.

One day, a pilot showed up to my office needing his medical. He was an established pilot with several hundred hours of flying, but he soon found himself embroiled in a quagmire of his own making.

He had been told by his own physician that he had diabetes and had been placed on medication, but it didn't occur to him to discuss this in advance with his new flight doctor. Instead, he chose a more common route. He showed up with documents from his physician describing his diabetes, as well as lab work showing he not only had diabetes, but that it wasn't really well controlled.

Now, the FAA does allow a lot of leeway for medication-controlled diabetics, and he was within their guidelines. But I informed him we would have to send all this info to the FAA and they would decide on his case. Unfortunately, it was a Saturday, so I wasn't able to call and get authorization that day, and he was leaving for a vacation the next week.

I began to tell him that I would fax it to them and then call them in a couple of days to get a verbal authorization, but he wasn't about to hear this.

He began complaining vigorously that he really didn't have diabetes and this was just a way to keep old pilots from flying. He wasn't really that old—not even in his seventies—so his complaint was comical in its naiveté.

So I showed him, using his own paperwork that he had brought to the exam, how he not only had diabetes, but that it wasn't even a close call;

he was clearly diabetic. This only upset the pilot further, and he became increasingly agitated, insisting that he certainly was not a diabetic.

Finally, despite my best calming efforts, he became so exasperated that he blurted out, "Well, I have a lot of other stuff, too, but I am not about to tell you about it!"

Now, laughing in his face wasn't an option—he might have suffered a heart attack or a stroke. Instead, I calmly explained that he was essentially admitting to a felony since he had sworn under penalty of perjury as to the accuracy of his health history, and that he likely would be permanently grounded until such time as the FAA allowed people to openly admit to perjury.

He calmed slightly and stated, "Well, I had leukemia, but I don't have to tell the FAA that!"

And by this time, I was temporarily questioning this whole pilot-referral concept.

▲ ▲ ▲

I encountered another referral when a very friendly pilot stated that he had a neighbor who was looking into becoming a pilot. The new applicant filled out his form and, as I reviewed it, I noted he had no surgical history and no other medical illnesses in his life. During the exam, however, as he removed his shirt, he revealed a massive abdominal scar.

"What occurred to cause that?" I asked.

"Oh, that was where I had my kidney removed."

Resisting the urge to ask if it were by magic, since he had reported no illnesses and no surgery, I asked, "What caused the kidney to need a removal?"

"Oh, I have cancer, but they removed it all."

So, by then I was a bit curious. "OK, did you bring me any records at all?"

"Oh, no. I don't need to do that. I don't have cancer anymore, so you can just give me my certificate."

This brings me to a new topic: naiveté and arrogance simply don't work well together. This gentleman, who was extremely wealthy and evidently used to getting his own way, refused to understand why a little doc-in-a-box flight surgeon would ever need to obtain records showing that he had been adequately treated, had fully followed up with his doctors, and had no residual cancer or metabolic issues related to losing a kidney. His word was sufficient to clear him, and that was going to be that. His disappointment led to him using some interesting descriptions of my lineage, which I didn't really find that insulting, since I had a pretty good grasp on my family tree.

This led me to wonder: when a person overreacts to a situation, is this often a sign of something deeper? That often seems to be the case. Overreactions are red flags to AMEs. Easy-to-spot red flags.

This gentleman isn't that rare, believe it or not. Many pilots go pretty far out of their way to downplay their medical conditions. A great many become incensed if you simply ask them for some records, when the condition wouldn't have been that big a hurdle to overcome. Ego, arrogance, and overreaction to minor issues are big red flags.

▲ ▲ ▲

Another day, a gentleman taking a variety of hormonal medications came in for a flight exam. He was a bit incensed when he heard that the FAA would want some paperwork on his recent pituitary gland surgery. He also was massively obese. He seemed upset that he would need to provide any documentation on a condition and a surgery that affected numerous pathways in his body, including his metabolism, kidney function, heart function, and so on.

That in and of itself was a bit strange. After all, the pituitary is essentially an extension of the brain within the skull. To make my point in as plain a way as possible, I pointed out to him that he had undergone brain surgery.

My thought was that *anyone* would realize this might be of concern to an agency monitoring pilot health, but at that point he blurted out, "But it was only a *small* brain surgery!"

I can proudly state that I repressed the strong urge to reply, "Obviously."

▲ ▲ ▲

Sometimes dragging the very basic info needed to make a decision can be painful.

"Any new medical issues?"

"I had a prostate biopsy."

"Why?"

"Don't know. My doctor said I needed it."

"What made him think you needed it?"

"I'm not sure?"

"Did you have an office visit, or did he just call you on the phone and say you needed a biopsy?"

"Oh, no. I went to his office, and he said I needed a biopsy."

"Did he do anything at all in the office during that visit? Tests? Blood work?"

"Oh, yeah, he did some blood work."

"What did the blood work show?"

"That I needed a biopsy, I guess."

There is a reason doctors ask patients to provide medical records.

▲ ▲ ▲

Sometimes the dishonesty of a pilot is a delayed response, but there are plenty of red flags in advance to make you think, *this is odd, nothing good will come of this.* Later, you realize why.

One day a gentleman called: "Hey, do you do ECGs?"

"Yes. Why? Do you need one?"

"Well, I am thinking about working on a flight medical later and want to do an ECG."

Now, this isn't usually something I'd do, but the guy talked me into it…or maybe it was a slow week or I was tired. The reason I don't do it is that half measures are usually half measures, and simply doing an ECG and nothing else on a patient isn't a test that brings a net positive result on average. After all, ECGs are terrible predictors of tomorrow.

My gut response should have been, "No, sir. Unless you are getting an FAA medical, there is zero utility to doing an ECG on a patient who has no symptoms that would make such a test appropriate."

But in a moment of weakness (or greed, who knows?) he was able to wheedle his way into a standalone ECG. A week later, dragging a huge backpack, appearing disheveled, smelling unkempt, and a veritable synonym soup of other homeless appellations, he showed up. He didn't look like a gentleman who would be able to afford basic flight training, and was near the borderline of being clinically diagnosable. But, he didn't quite totally cross the barrier, and I was only doing an ECG. (See how powerful rationalization can be? I knew something wasn't fitting, but I talked myself into doing the ECG.)

So I did it, gave him a copy, scanned another copy into my computer, and off he went. His explanation was, "I wanted to make sure my ECG was going to be good, because I heard that was needed." He also stated that he had taken some flight lessons years before and thought maybe he'd switch careers.

Six months later, I get a phone call from the same gentleman. He is at a flight school and wants me to fax him over a copy of the *medical certificate* that I did on him six months prior. This incredible gentleman apparently thought I was going to completely forget this singular incident of an apparent homeless man who hadn't apparently bathed within the past century and who was on the border of mental illness, showing up for only an ECG. He also apparently thought that this doctor with no memory could be talked into issuing him a medical certificate when he'd never had any medical exam performed.

I've not figured out if this was an incredibly well thought out but completely stupid plan (the exams are stored in a computer database, it's almost impossible to pretend you had an exam if you didn't have one). Or perhaps he was a mentally ill or drugged person who forgot that he'd repeatedly called my office to set up *just* an ECG, and then while he was lying on my exam table having the ECG done, talked in detail about why he only wanted an ECG.

▲ ▲ ▲

The concept of downplaying a current medical condition is understandable. However, sometimes a person will downplay a condition to the extent of absurdity. One day, a longtime pilot came to my office in full flight uniform. The pilot was limping severely, so I asked him what was wrong.

"Doc, my sciatica is killing me."

"Well, what are you doing here?"

"I need my flight exam. I have to fly out today."

Luckily, I knew the pilot and was able to laugh at his poor judgment while comically pointing out to him at least one possible issue he might not have thought about relating to him heading off to the airport.

"Really," I said. "Hey, let me ask you a question. Besides pilots and passengers, do FAA personnel ever go to airports?"

"Yep."

"And do they ever check medicals?"

"Yep."

"So, to be clear, you want to limp through the center of two of the busiest airports in the world today—with my name on your certificate *signed today,* stating that you are safe to fly—while you drag your leg past thousands of passengers and numerous FAA personnel tasked with preventing a safety issue from occurring. Is that the basic concept?"

This pilot had the ability to see the absurdity of his decision-making. He called later and apologized for not thinking about the situation. He ended up either having lower back surgery or removing his oversized wallet from his back pocket and went back to flying soon thereafter.

It is very nice when a pilot realizes his judgment was the issue and that the AME wasn't just being arbitrary.

▲ ▲ ▲

Another gentleman wasn't so understanding—after all, he'd driven an hour to get here, then showed up with an actively flaring gouty toe and limped into my office.

"Come back after the gout flare is gone," I said.

"But I drove an hour to get here!"

Finesse required. "I can't certify you to fly if you aren't fit to fly."

"But it will be gone soon."

A lesser man would become frustrated. Hell, who am I kidding? I *am* a lesser man, and I began to get frustrated, but I finally convinced him that a flight doctor would be a really stupid flight doctor to certify a guy who limps into his office in severe pain. But I have to tell you, it took a lot of talking.

And that should scare most folks with a little bit of intelligence.

▲ ▲ ▲

One of my all-time favorites has so many elements of comedy to it that it still stands out in my mind.

Whunk, whunk, whunk. Up the steps I can heard what sounded like a man on crutches. I thought, *If this guy is here for a flight physical, I am going to be ticked.* This was unusual, as my anger usually doesn't exhibit a clarity of prescience before it arrives on scene. But—around the corner came a man on crutches, with a leg cast up to the knee.

"I am here to get a flight physical."

"Why are you on crutches and in a cast?"

"I had my Achilles tendon repaired this week and I have a couple weeks off, so I want to go flying."

Later that same week:

"Hey John, this is Dave over at the airport. Did some guy in crutches come in there?"

"Yep. Are you to blame for that?"

"Oh, no. We told him he couldn't rent an airplane because he couldn't pass a medical, and he said, 'Oh yeah? Well, I'll be right back. I am going to find a flight doctor to pass me.'"

Over time, I forgot all about this incident, except when I might have wanted to have a good laugh. Five years later I was in a new office on the other side of town, and I am by then eighty pounds lighter.

One day, a gentleman walked in. His certificate was seven years out of date, which isn't that rare, but I do think of this as an occasional red flag. He wanted to get back into flying.

"What happened to make you stop flying?" (It's a great question to find out underlying medical issues, by the way.)

"Well, doc, I kind of got discouraged, because I went to this doctor up on Colonial Drive and he threw me out of his office."

"Why?"

"Well, I had torn my Achilles tendon, and I just dropped in to ask him when he thought it might be safe to go back. You know, I think he just totally misunderstood me..."

Hmm, knowing the backstory, I had a feeling I didn't misunderstand him then, and I wasn't misunderstanding him now.

▲ ▲ ▲

Sometimes, the first-time medical problem doesn't even occur in the flight doctor's office. Pilots often get into trouble simply because they've really never had any medical issues crop up in the past. They will assume an air of invincibility that is only shattered when they are faced with a new medical condition...or in some cases, a hilarious chain of events, such as this case.

The typical pilot may stop by a mall on the way to work with a couple of hours to kill before a flight, and they may just stroll around looking for special deals. They do have a reputation to uphold for being (*ahem*) cost conscious. But one story resonated with me more than others.

"Reza" was walking through a mall and saw an advertisement by a chiropractor for a chair massage for just twenty-five dollars. He'd only just gotten to the mall though, so he decided to keep strolling; he had some time to kill. Later he came across an optometrist office advertising eye exams. The cost seemed very cheap, so he said to himself, "Well, after all, I am forty years old. I've never been to an eye doctor, so this is a great idea."

He entered the optometrist's lair and sat in the exam chair while the assistant explained to him all the details of an eye exam. He, however, was thinking about his flight to Quito.

"Tilt your head back," she said. "We are going to put some drops in your eyes so that we can see your eyes more clearly." So back went his head, and he sat there while the optometrist entered and introduced himself.

Reza was a nervous sort, a guy with "white-coat hypertension" who gets excited even if a family member takes his blood pressure. He got a little unnerved when the optometrist said, "Well, it's still a bit hard to see back there, but let's give it thirty minutes for the drops to work, and then we'll take another look."

So Reza went off strolling through the mall. Then he was struck by an inspiration: "Hey, this is just enough time to get that chair massage!" And off he went.

About fifteen minutes into the chair massage, he opened his eyes and everything was blurry. He panicked and began asking the massage therapist what she has done to cause his vision to blur. She freaked out because she has only been massaging his neck. They started getting upset with each other until he decided to call his girlfriend, who works at a doctor's office.

"Honey, I am getting a massage, and my vision just went all blurry."

Now his girlfriend was all upset, because she thought he was headed to the airport, and here he is, telling her he's getting a massage. After a bit of back-and-forth and explaining profusely, Reza calmed her down.

She asked him about anything else he was doing that afternoon, and he told her about the eye exam.

"Wait! Did they put any drops in your eyes?"

He paused, sensing a trap. "Well, yeah…they said it would make it easier to see."

Thunk, thunk, thunk went her head on the desk.

"Reza! They dilated your eyes!"

He had never heard of such a thing. "They did what to my eyes?"

So she explained how dilating eyes works, and by now he was *really* upset because he had an hour before he needed to get to the airport and two hours before takeoff. The massage therapist had to guide him back to the optometrist because he was half blind and couldn't even remember where the place was. Now the doctor began trying to calm him down.

"Sir, I understand you have a flight; don't worry, this will wear off in a day at the most. You will be fine. Just sit back and have a cocktail and enjoy the flight."

"But sir…I am the pilot!"

At this point, the optometrist got nervous and said, "Oh, well, it'll probably wear off in a couple of hours."

11

The Light Casualty Class of Aircraft

or, Why Can Grandpa Fly His Cub When He Can't Tie My Shoe?

So, BACK TO the FAA and being careful not to bite the hand that feeds too much. If you do, use a mild pepper in your condiments; ghost peppers can really linger. Let's talk about the light-sport fiasco.

In about 2004 or so, the FAA came up with the light-sport category after a lot of back and forth with so-called stakeholders. These folks collect monies from pilots to create a niche profession and then pretend to advocate in all manners of conflicting manners both for pilot safety and the equally reverse concept of total lack of pilot responsibility…and yes, I do include the AOPA in this group. We'll talk more on the third-party leech system later. Frankly, to my slanted view, this decision by the FAA was a cynical way of saying, *Hey, let's get rid of our sickest patients…let's let them become a high-risk legal pool.*

Now, I don't want to bore you with detail on who, what, where, or why, but the classification is for small planes doing daytime flying with limited seats. It was also meant to put stronger oversight above the ultralight group of planes while allowing older, diseased pilots with marked health issues to forego getting a medical and to kill themselves with a less complex and, in some cases, slower vehicle.

In other words, they designed a lawyer's dream: a class so full of suit opportunity that you could float a seaplane on the legal drool that pooled around. Several lawyers even stopped chasing ambulances and began barking at passing ice cream trucks...but that metaphor really seems not to work here. *Hmm.*

But I am being metaphorical, perhaps not well. The light-sport class made no sense at all, but it was what it was. Around 2011, an AOPA writer noted that accident rates were about three times as common as in general aviation...but that was OK, because the FAA didn't design the class to be safer than GA (which already has a relatively high accident rate). No, it had designed the light-sport class to be safer than the ultralight class. I had to applaud the spin this AOPA writer put on the stats.

Later, other AOPA writers who simply made up facts such as, "no light-sport accident has ever been tied to a probable medical incapacitation," buried those stats under myth and legend. I found ten accidents in fewer than five minutes that had occurred well before he wrote the article and that he should have known about with the most basic of research—all on the NTSB website and all within a few months of one another.

But why was the LSA class a bad idea in the first place?

Well, for one, by getting rid of the medical, you put a bunch of people into the sky who had already stopped flying because of medical issues, but now, without the FAA looking on and with their delusions of former competence or even former sanity, these folks took to the sky. I, unlike AOPA, don't mind citing accidents specifics: one had a seizure history, another had severe heart disease and was on several conflicting antidepressants as well as antianxiolytics *and* a sleeping pill that was also in the antianxiolytic class. If you don't believe me, it's on the NTSB accident searchable database. Look up the last three months of 2013. The GA accident fatality reports there aren't that flattering either.

But the other thing the FAA did was allow people to lapse their third-class special issuance and let them move to light sport with known issues and no FAA oversight. This is especially troubling when you read what the first paragraph of a special-issuance letter says, "We have decided you have a medical condition that you shouldn't legally be able to fly on…unless you have oversight."

I'm paraphrasing, but if that is true, then pilots with third-class medicals today have to have this letter, yet a pilot in the LSA class with a known same condition doesn't. The FAA is saying that they are creating a class wherein they will allow people to fly when they already know for a fact these people shouldn't be flying without oversight. Nevertheless, what the heck, go for it.

This becomes logically ridiculous. A special-issuance condition is put in place to allow pilots to fly despite a known dangerous medical condition that could affect safe operation of aircraft. It allows a person to fly anyway, as long as oversight is in place. Now, however, we are going to allow this person to knowingly lapse the certificate and then to continue to fly with a known condition that is incompatible with flight.

Thunk, thunk, thunk.

Meanwhile, the FAA has also created a class where myths can begin, where pilots create a mythology that they are just as safe as GA. This class adopts as its white knight a guy who can't see an X on a runway with construction equipment all over it. This guy can land on the closed runway anyway and then lie to the FAA and then get so irate about the situation that he can get a bill put up to do away with all third-class medicals, using a cynical misinformation campaign based upon an entire stack of lies and myths and nonexistent statistics.

Thunk, thunk, thunk.

You can bet the deaf, blind guy would have loved to have had the light-sport option, and he'd have taken his mobile home to the airfield at least once, provided he made it there alive.

12

What if You Commit a Crime and No One Wants to Help?

or, Doc, You Are so Uncooperative—Don't You Want to Be Roommates in Federal Prison?

IN MY EXPERIENCE, a subset of pilots routinely makes totally selfish, totally immature decisions and knowingly flies when they and their families as well are well aware that they have no business flying. Let me repeat the operative word: *routinely*.

But worse is the pilot who then tries to coerce the AME to violate federal law. These people often haven't even been to the AME they are attempting to engage in conspiracy. And it happens so much that it is why I formulated my three rules.

These three rules exist precisely because of how often they are violated. They are: (1) don't show up sick; (2) if you have a new condition, let me know about it as early in advance of your exam as possible (with two exceptions we will see later); and (3) don't ask me to do anything illegal. You've heard this before, but it bears a lot of repeating.

The fact that these three rules are the most common mistakes pilots make (and they make them at least weekly at my practice) should be enough for an *honest* aviation writer to admit that maybe some of the aviation bloggers have become simply mouthpieces for an agenda and have lost all sense of objectivity. After all, if pilots routinely show up for flight medicals sick or asking to do things that aren't legal or with new conditions they haven't bothered to find out are grounding conditions, then aren't these pilots also flying?

It is a rhetorical question, because they all certify how many hours they flew in the past six months, and in the vast majority of these very common incidents, the pilot will have logged a lot of hours during that same time they were admitting to having grounding conditions (rule two). Often they fly with conditions that they wish the doctor to conceal from the FAA (the very common violation of rule number three).

The methodology of coercion is often hilariously childish.

A patient with occasional bouts of atrial fibrillation will say to an AME (it has happened to me more than once): "Hey, doc. Off the record, I've had some A-fib, but it is all gone, so, that's off the record."

That's really comical, since I haven't worked for a newspaper in over twenty years, and then it was only writing local sports copy. "Off the record" is easy to interpret. It really means: "Hey, doc, would you please commit a federal felony for me?" Of course they don't ask that outright for some reason. Puzzling.

Another phrase used quite often is: "Don't tell them, but..." That explains my new baseball cap with the bill that reads: "but, but, but...I am them."

Paranoid pilots are the ones who ask the most silly of things on the phone and via e-mail. I remember one pilot with a nonmetastic type of skin cancer that was really nothing at all to be too worried about; in fact, the FAA had just changed its standards regarding this localized skin cancer. But this pilot was really paranoid. In prior visits he had talked about how NSA is watching everyone, how he felt that government was overreaching into all aspects of life...

Of course, he is correct in some regards, but that doesn't make his story less fun to tell. A few months after his visit, he called up to tell me he has skin cancer.

"Hey, doc, I remember you told me to call you ASAP if anything new happens. Well, I got a skin cancer." He described which type.

I was happy he followed my rules, and I proceeded to thank him. Then I said, "Look, this is no biggie; send me the reports, and I'll forward them to the FAA." (At the time, the FAA was requesting BCC or SCC reports for this type of cancer; they don't now.)

So he then said, "Well, I don't want you to tell them that."

"I can't not tell them; if I withhold the information for you, you are asking me to commit a crime."

"I think you are overreacting," he said.

"You think I am overreacting. I want to make sure the FAA doesn't accuse me of underreacting. They're the ones listening in on this phone call right now, according to you, buddy, so unless you were lying to me last week about them recording all our conversations, I am not about to underreact when I know what their policies are."

The phone went silent for a bit…then *click, buzz*.

He called back a while later. He was a bit calmer and ready to be reassured that telling the FAA information about a completely resolved insignificant issue wasn't a huge conspiracy.

▲ ▲ ▲

A different pilot e-mailed me: "I am also a health-care provider. I need a flight exam." I told him about my website where he can make an appointment.

He e-mailed me again: "I am also a health-care provider. I need a flight exam."

I by then am thinking to myself—and trust me, that isn't what you want me doing—so I e-mailed him back: "Our website is […]. We have an online appointment system; you can make an appointment based upon your schedule there. Also, what medical issues do you have?"

He e-mailed me back and told me some of medical issues he has had. I advise him that he needs to bring A, B, C, D, and E documents. He shows up with A, B, C, and D, but no E.

And so off he went grumbling, and a week or so later he came back with A, B, C, D, and E documents. I reviewed them all, and he's fine. The world is at peace; birds chirp; the clouds clear…

And then I began his exam, and me being me and him being an American (and by that I do mean obese), I, as a joke, asked this pilot who has been getting medicals for years from other doctors, "So how long you been on a CPAP machine?"

"Oh, about fifteen years."

Thunk, thunk, thunk went my head on the wall. This guy fell for the oldest trick in the book—he thought I heard something in his lungs, so cue the reversion to honesty. I catch a lot of smokers by asking them how much they smoke while I am examining their ears.

I explained to him that we now needed documents F, G, and H, and he got all upset again. "But, doc, I didn't put it because there was no place on the forms for sleep apnea."

I pointed out that his argument is a bit flawed because sleep apnea has been a huge and very contentious topic with the FAA for the past several years, as AOPA, ALPA, EAA, and the federal air surgeon or someone at the FAA had ham-handed this issue into the ground through misstep after hilarious misstep. It was a bit like watching two autonomous robots playing tennis with an anvil…entertaining, but they really chunk up the landscape.

But I digress—his argument was flawed because he had used the other illness box to report other issues, so he knew the box existed. Added to that, the gentleman had not reported it for the past fifteen years. So I had to wonder—it never occurred to this "health professional" to report his sleep apnea on any of those multiple exams?

More importantly, and I promise a whole chapter on red flags, what he didn't know was that I had been watching him like a hawk from the get-go because he had already red flagged himself as a suspicious character. After all, what do I care if he was another healthcare professional; yet, he sure wanted me to know it. He had been red-flag material from his very first e-mail.

Anyway, I bandaged and stitched my scalp from having banged it on the wall, and off he went.

The next day, he e-mailed me: "You and I are the only ones who know I am on a CPAP. Why Don't we just not tell the FAA, and we go ahead and issue me a certificate?"

"HAHAHAHAAHA" This is my memory of the sounds occurring as I rolled on the floor.

So I e-mailed him back after significantly pausing to reflect, rewrite, and thank computer designers for making keyboards that can sustain head blows.

"Sir, overlooking your improper use of the pronoun we, you have asked me to commit a federal crime. Now, I am a fairly reasonable guy, so do me a favor, so that I am not simply confused. Resend me the same message, but in the subject line please type: DEAR DOCTOR SHEWMAKER, I WOULD LIKE YOU TO COMMIT A FEDERAL CRIME."

Then I hit SEND and waited for his e-mail to come back.

"Oh, I would never ask you to do anything to put your license in jeopardy; after all, I am also in the health-care field." I experienced a visceral urge to type, "Do you mean twice?" But I refrained. (And by that I mean, I may have typed it, but I didn't send it.)

▲ ▲ ▲

On the rule about coming to the office sick: One day, I was reviewing the office rules with a couple of pilots in the lobby. I tried to do this in pairs so that people can discuss the rules. This helps make sure it sticks in the pilots' minds a bit longer. Anyway, I get to the rule about not coming to the exam sick, and one of the pilots, who seen me several times, turned to the other pilot who was new, and said, "He is serious. I did it once, and he threw me out."

▲ ▲ ▲

Speaking of a person using their employment as a coercive tool, one day a pilot walked in, slammed his paperwork on the counter, and rudely yelled, "I have an appointment." He claimed he had no medical issues and signed his name to the form under penalty of perjury. I let him stand there for a few seconds as a test to see if he was routinely a rude jerk or to see if this was a momentary reaction to other events. He began drumming his fingers.

"So, no medical issues?"

"No. Look, I have been in the military. I have served my country. I have doctors at the VA. What do I need this for?"

"I understand this seems a bit redundant, sir, but we'll get you taken care of."

And so I continued with some computer work for ten or fifteen seconds, just to continue seeing his reaction. I was rapidly becoming convinced he was a sociopath.

"Ever had surgery?"

"Maybe." Turns out, he hadn't just lied about surgery, he was also being treated for a variety of things, and when I asked him why he didn't put them on the form he'd sworn was accurate, he stated, "If I wrote down all my issues, I'd have to write a book."

So, in the course of three minutes, this person admitted he had committed a federal crime simply because he was too lazy to type in all his medical issues. And this was totally predictable, based upon his first three seconds in the office. It turns out, that was just the tip of Mr. Iceberg's problems.

Of course, this begs the question, how do some persons get such a sense of audacity and lose their entire sense of judgment to attempt such a brazen act as to coerce an FAA designated and trained AME into a criminal conspiracy, or to think that a professional medical examiner won't notice their obvious dishonesty? I think the answer is very simple, very complicated, and extremely illustrative.

I think it is because, for many years, pilots have specifically sought out AMEs who will pass a sea slug with an AmEx card, pulse optional. So then, many pilots really expect that AMEs who have a reputation of being helpful to pilots will also then be helpful to criminal pilots. To these pilots, "helpful" is code for "criminal conspirator." I believe this is a decades-long evolutionary process, and I think members of the FAA are fully aware of the issue. In fact, they work very hard at trying to figure out how to stop it, all the while missing how easy it would be to fix it.

13

But This Isn't Judgment Day

or, Judgment? We Don't Need No Stinkin' Judgment!

A LOT OF THE anecdotes that occur in my office revolve around just basic, simple, bad judgment. Mine for answering the phone when I am in the middle of something else isn't included here, but it is rare that good comes from that event.

There are four main points to know here: (1) these types of events happen weekly; (2) people with an agenda are out there claiming these folks should be able to fly on a driver's license; (3) no one believes the DMV does a good job vetting drivers; and (4) accident rates don't improve by reducing safety screening. So here are some examples.

Eighty-two-year-old, healthy-as-a-horse guy called up. "I want to renew me a flight exam." (He sounded like a hoarse Sam Elliot speaking through a paper-towel roll in a tunnel with marbles in his mouth.)

I asked him if he has any medical problems.

"Nope. I am healthy as a horse. Never been sick." I told him about the MedXPress form he needed to complete. He called back two weeks later, and I asked again (knowing already it is the same voice I am hearing), if he has any medical problems.

"Nope, I'm healthy as a horse!" I asked about his last doctor visit. "Never been sick; been twenty years or more since I saw a doctor, I haven't been sick a day in my life." So I asked for his date of birth to check to see if there is anything in the scant info the FAA website allows me to find, and he said, "I am eighty-two years old."

I asked him, "You have *never* had anything? No skin issues, prostate issue, colonoscopy?"

"Well now, I did have a few skin cancers taken off a while back, but that's just the sun damage. No big thing."

"When was that, sir?"

"Well, let's see…that would have been five years ago, before my heart stents."

Thunk, thunk, thunk, thunk, thunk.

▲ ▲ ▲

A pilot marked all no's on his form. I listened to his heart—I actually felt the heave and then listened for the murmur. He was a thin twenty-four-year-old; this could be functional, but it was a pretty good heave. He told me, "Well, they knew about the murmur on my European flight physical, and I had a full work-up."

"OK, but no paperwork?"

"But they said I was OK."

"You mean those people who regulate pilots in a different country than the United States?" *Hmm.*

▲ ▲ ▲

This one happens at least ten times a year. Pilot showed up on Saturday and said, "My ALPA doc says you can pass me." Then the pilot plopped down a hundred pages on my desk.

"When did you have your issue?" I asked.

"Oh, about eight months ago."

"Well, since you think eight months is a good enough length of time to wait before telling me, come back in eight months after I have had time to read this novel. That way, the other ten people waiting to see me today aren't impacted."

OK, maybe I just thought that. Instead, I said, "Well, we need to schedule you for a time the FAA is open, because it's Saturday."

▲ ▲ ▲

This one happens five times a year at a minimum. Guy showed up at six o'clock. FAA in Oklahoma City closed at five thirty our time.

"I talked to my AOPA people, and they said all you have to do is call the FAA, and you can pass me."

"Did you bring me anything to look at? Reports?"

"Oh, no…they're handling that."

So, the FAA is closed, I have nothing to discuss with them, and the pilot got mad at me because some third party told him to come see me without a pre-exam call.

▲ ▲ ▲

ADHD guy walked out of the office, leaving his wallet on the table.

As a joke, I asked him, "So, how long have you had ADHD?"

He said, "Ha-ha, that's a trick question."

"Why?"

"I have had it my whole life," he says. "You are born with it."

▲ ▲ ▲

Flight instructors who don't tell their pilot applicants to get their medical at hour one instead of the night before their solo…*grrrrr*…they provide anger management testing. It usually takes two to three months to solo, but only five to six weeks to clear a medical issue with the FAA. You can train while you are getting medically cleared—but you can't solo if you are not cleared medically. Come in early!

▲ ▲ ▲

A pilot showed up in full-blown delusional crisis. I sent him off to the psych ward. It's not a daily occurrence, but it has happened. And when you are legally committing people on the day they choose to get a flight medical, you stop and think. *Hmm.*

▲ ▲ ▲

"Does the FAA want all my DUIs or just my last one?"
"How many DUIs have you had, sir?"
The answer was a puzzled look followed by, "I don't really know."

▲ ▲ ▲

A pilot marked all no's on the form, but the moment we got in the exam room, he told me about his testicular cancer that had also possibly spread to his lungs.
"But I am cured now, doc." No doctor's letters, no hospital notes; I'm just supposed to take his word for it.

▲ ▲ ▲

Pilot walked in for the tenth time in ten years, and once again had brought some of his glaucoma reports but not all. I called over to his doctor, who agreed to fax over the rest. Instead (and this happens three or four times a year), the office faxes over his entire record…and that was how his diabetes that he had been lying about for years got reported to the FAA. I gave him a bulleted list of instructions, including that he has to wait sixty days and redo blood work, because he'd stopped his medication for several months just before coming to the exam.

Now, what did he do? He didn't follow directions; he called me weekly to whine about how if his lab values had been a tiny bit better, this wouldn't have mattered, and (despite my constant reminder that it was only his stopping his meds and his dishonesty that had caused his issue) this went on for months.

To this day, he proclaims to all in earshot how the bad FAA people wouldn't let his dishonest butt get into an airplane until he had met their previously published guidelines that he could have read at any time during the ten years he had very well-controlled diabetes and chose to lie about it. Then decided to stop his medications. And then once again forgot his visual fields. That led to a nurse violating federal HIPAA laws by sending over the wrong records with no signed release to another physician…who then found out that the pilot had a ten-year track record of felonious actions.

But the FAA was the bad guy? The delusion is strong in this one!

▲ ▲ ▲

Sometimes, you figure out that the FAA does have a good reason for some of the things you might think are somewhat silly. This happened to me with two incidents that occurred in close proximity.

The FAA says that you need to have a device to occlude the eyes. Well, me being a rational thinker, I figured to myself that a hand is a device, and a hand is opaque, so a hand legally fits this requirement. In fact, a hand doesn't do the trick, and you should not use a hand.

Why? Well, pilot number one had 20/20 vision standing up, then as I was standing above him while he looked into the keystone telebinocular (this machine gets some fun incidents), instead of putting his head into the headrest, he put his head so that his right eye can look into the left eyehole. I made him place his head properly, and he failed miserably in—wait for it—his left eye. This guy knew for four months he had an eye issue and didn't fix it. Another guy, a foreign pilot, knew he had a severe cataract, yet he flew over and tried to get his exam. But he didn't cheat; he just didn't fix the problem when he should have done so.

▲ ▲ ▲

Another eye incident really illustrates the hand problem, as well as the pathetic nature of a liar caught in the lie. This guy has 20/20 in his left eye, then put his head into the machine for near vision and was stone cold 20/100 on the left.

I find this weird and asked him, "So why didn't you bring glasses?" Well, the doc told him glasses wouldn't work because he has amblyopia. "That affects your distant vision as well, right?"

He said yes, so I asked how he got 20/20 on the distant vision (knowing he cheated, obviously). He said, "I don't know, maybe the light was coming in between my fingers a bit."

Thunk, thunk, thunk.

▲ ▲ ▲

Another gentleman came in and tried to look with his left eye into the right eye slot on the near-vision machine and then when I busted him on this fraud, stated, "Oh, yeah, I knew I had a problem. I saw an eye doctor in January about it." It was July, and he had simply ignored a potential flight hazard issue and then tried to fake his way through his exam.

▲ ▲ ▲

Yet another guy came in with severe cataracts. He'd flown into the country just to get his flight medical, knowing he was blind in one eye; yet he pretended to be shocked that this would be considered an issue. In the course of his repeated rationalizations for ignoring his cataract, however, he inadvertently admitted that other doctors had advised him that this might be a problem he should fix prior to his flight exam.

▲ ▲ ▲

Sometimes it is a flight school that does something amazingly obtuse. One flight school was famous for overworking its instructors. One instructor fell asleep while leaving his facility at 2:00 a.m. and ran into the side of a hangar with his car. Immediately, they sent him to their favorite AME who evaluated him, said he was fine, and sent him back.

This was not good enough for them, so they insisted that he see a neurologist. Off he went, had a long evaluation, and passed. They still weren't happy; they thought that seemed too easy, so then they sent him to another AME—and that was me.

He told his story to me, who had once watched a movie called *Death on the Highway* as an eighth grader and who himself once fell asleep after working two or three shifts while in college and ran into the back of a car at a red light.

I listened to his story, chuckled, and told him that the cure to being sleepy is, quite amazingly, sleep. So I passed him—he had no issues, no red flags at all, and off he went.

One day later the flight school called: "Dr. Shewmaker, are you sure he is OK to fly?"

"You are asking me, the AME, who is tasked with deciding whether he is OK to fly?"

"Yes, we are asking you."

"Definitely, he is very good to go."

"How can you tell?"

"It's my job."

"Don't you need to do more testing?"

"On him or on you?" (I just thought this.) Aloud, I said, "Look, since the flight doctor's opinion, the second flight doctor's opinion, and the neurologist's opinion don't seem to match your higher degree of medical training, I will tell you what. I will call up the AMCD doctors and explain the details, OK?" I may have been slightly nicer in my tone/verbiage.

"Oh, OK, Thanks."

One minute into my hilarious conversation with the AMCD doctor, I am trying to be totally serious while listening to the following: "He fell asleep? At two in the morning? After working all day and night? Well, what do you want to know? He was tired! It's called sleeping! He is OK, Dr. Shewmaker!"

So I hung up the phone, knowing my reputation is never going to recover from that phone call, and I called the flight school back. "I talked to the FAA medical staff, they said he is OK."

"Are you sure?"

"Yep."

"He doesn't need more testing?"

"I might wanna test his decision-making when it comes to flight school choices." (No, I didn't say it.)

"Hang on. I want to get the VP on the phone."

"Sure, but I gotta tell you, I am getting sleepy." (Again, didn't say it.)

"Dr. Shewmaker, we are really concerned here. This guy fell asleep when he was driving, and you are saying you can't do anything further to evaluate this?"

There is a bit of a limit to my patience, and I was way past its normal breaking point. For some reason I hadn't hung up on them yet…but it was time.

"Here's a freaking test for you. Stop violating federal employment law by forcing people to work sixteen to eighteen hours a day for six days a week without proper reimbursement under the guise of volunteer work and do that for six months and see how many incidents happen then, buddy. Because your false pretense of giving a crap about safety ignores the salient point that his episode of falling asleep is a part of the endemic culture you have set up. Sleeping is a normal physiological response to fatigue, just as hanging up is a normal physiological response to having heard enough bullshit to last a lifetime." (That may not be verbatim.)

One really has to wonder what motivates a person to come to an exam with a known medical condition and attempt to fake their way through the exam. But I am going to stop this chapter now, because judgment could be a book all on its own, and I have way too many of these stories to tell in just one chapter. So let's divvy them up.

14

Is That a Pet Peeve, or Are You Just Way Too Sensitive?

or, If You Hear It Enough, You'll Go Blind

SOME OF THE enjoyable parts of my job are those daily events that make me laugh at my own foibles. I have always been a little self-absorbed and a little vain and a little too focused on finishing the job.

This predilection for peevishness has often led me to declare that I am going to post my lists of pet peeves on my door, but then I quickly developed two new pet peeves. It peeved me that I couldn't put my pet peeves on the door, and it peeved me that my door was too small for them all. Thankfully, these are more like minor irritations that I have learned to recognize, to look for, and to laugh at myself for, over and over. Sometimes they do get me into trouble, especially when enough of them occur in a short enough time that I don't realize my minor irritations are piling up, and then I overreact inappropriately to a situation. Usually, though, it is the actual situation that causes the reaction—and usually the reaction is to intentionally *underreact* to some silliness a patient has decided to perpetrate.

I like bulleted lists, so here are some examples of the petty, daily irritants that remind me to laugh at myself.

- Five times a day, I hear, "Doc, my middle name is all lowercased, but the rest of my name is all capitalized." (The MedXPress system does this, and it does looks weird.) I sigh and explain that, yep, that's just how the system is. But it does cause a little, internal urge to let out a primal scream sometimes.
- Pilots who will not leave their heads in the machine for near vision until all five of the cards are read. I am trying to do their vision testing, and they are bobbing back and forth like that old cracker-barrel sipping bird.
- Pilots who look at the eye chart endlessly but don't say anything. Then, after what seems like hours of staring, pull out their glasses and say, "Oh, that's better."
- Pilots who are five minutes late on the last appointment of the day, especially on Friday. Also, those who are late on the first exam of the day.
- Pilots who will see that you have five people in the lobby, and decide to engage you in endless, irrelevant, small talk.
- Pilots who hand you thirty pages to read and then ask you unrelated questions while you are trying to do so.
- Pilots who walk up to you while carrying a cup of urine with no cap placed upon it, having traversed carpet and say, "I tried to fill it as full as possible."
- People who show up early and then sit in the parking lot instead of coming in to see if you are ready to get their exam done. A variation is when they also have thirty pages of new medical information but sit in the car instead of getting it into your hands.
- People who will stand in front of you with thirty pages of medical records and attempt to slowly describe random details in the records instead of handing them to you so you can start determining the options available. Sometimes, I just grab the pages out of their hands, and if they start to protest, I tell them, "Hush. I am reading this so that I can help you." We can all be our own worst enemies.

- People who say that they are six feet tall. And then they just have to say it…. "That's seventy-two inches". Thunk, Thunk, Thunk.
- People who ask what form of payment I prefer and then pay with the only thing they brought. "What payment do you prefer?"
    "Cash."
    "Oh, well…all I brought was a check [credit card, baked pie, etc.]."
- Bathing. This is simply rude. People who had plenty of time to bathe but show up smelling like a goat get my radar going. If they aren't paying attention to their body odor and its impact on other people, what else does this possibly mean?
- Smokers who stand right outside then walk in, reeking. I usually make them come back in fifteen minutes and tell them it is because I want their BP to normalize. And by *their*, I mean *mine*.
- People who say while doing the eye chart: P, E, Zulu, maybe an O, L, Charlie, F, either a T or a Q, Delta. OK, look. Choose a method—letters or phonetic—and tell me what you see. Either you missed it or maybe you missed it. Say the letters and let the chips fall, but don't try to give me a seizure by switching back and forth between A, Bravo, C, Delta, E, Foxtrot. There isn't enough Tylenol in the world for the headache that gives me.
- *Hmm.* I think listing my pet peeves is a new pet peeve for me. This listing is starting to irritate me.
- People who stand outside, never checking the door to see if it is unlocked. Instead, they knock incessantly or open the door a crack and yell "Hellooo!" into the door or call on the phone—in front of an unlocked door!—and ask if you are open.
- Foreign pilots who question you repeatedly if their height and weight is correct after you just weighed them and they were facing the scale reading and you showed them that in the English measuring system, they were X pounds and Y inches. And then they ask what that is in kilograms. I always laugh and say, easier math.

- ⏱ Obese pilots who refuse to answer your trap question: "So, what is your biggest issue that you think can affect your health?" Don't be coy; the elephant in the room isn't going to disappear. It's your obesity.

    I just want to hear you say it. (See the chapter on obesity.)

I could go on and on, but this chapter was just filler to get you to buy the book; after all, I can't sell you a seventy-page book. I gotta flesh it out. That is also the reason for the slightly larger font and the pinched margins, but, hey, you are fourteen chapters in, might as well finish.

After all, aren't you also all about finishing the job?

15

Assorted Red Flags

or, You Told Me a Lot and Didn't Say Anything at All

Throughout this book, I have mentioned various red flags. In this chapter, I've gathered a great collection of short little red-flag statements. Many of these are obvious; some are subtle.

- When a person calls for you by name or insists on speaking directly to the doctor instead of talking to whoever answers. Look:You don't know me, and you are calling a doctor's office. Don't pretend you know me, and don't pretend your issues are so earth-shattering that I need to drop everything I am doing with my scheduled appointments to speak with you. An honest broker would say, "Can Dr. Shewmaker call me about a question I have?" But "Is John there?" tells me I can bet coercion is right around the corner.
- When a person shows up with no ID.
- When a person who is from another country gets upset with you because they have no ID on them.
- When a spouse or partner stands right next to the person during the entire exam.
- When a person goes out of their way to tell you they are also in the medical profession. Repeatedly.

- When a wife calls for a husband or vice versa.
- Trembling hands—not that uncommon, and often caused by reasons other than just a normal tremor.
- Sweating.
- Becoming argumentative.
- Attempting to pee on the trees in my territory. The pilot who begins asserting dominance from the moment he enters almost always has something wrong and is attempting intimidation. That, of course, is always a source of laughter, since you can't intimidate the guy who pushes the Print Certificate button. You are playing draw poker in a tank top with a magician; the intimidation game isn't ever gonna work. All you will do is fail your exam, while you go away thinking, *Wow, that was such a nice gentle doctor. He spent so much time softly explaining to me how I wasn't going to fly today.*

    It is totally optional whether I call AMCD and obtain your special issuance on day one or whether I let them handle it over the next six weeks. At the end of the day, I have four royal flushes and thirty-two other cards on my side of the table. I have already won the intimidation game, so it bores me to even bother with it. I win. When you come to me, you will get the same treatment as every other person, no matter what. There is no other level of mocking higher than that to a person who thinks their expelled waste doesn't stink. If this is still your style, then you don't understand what I just wrote. Intimidation is comical, and depending on the AME you go to, it may just cost you about six weeks of pay. On the other hand, knowing your position in the pecking order might just result in you losing no money at all. It's something to consider.

    But I am writing this for the 90 percent of pilots who won't try this tactic; the ones who would try intimidation already know everything about everything, so they aren't reading this anyway.
- People who negate their processes. "I have a tiny bit of diabetes," "I had a small penis infection," etc.
- Those who show up with their urine already in a cup.

- When a person faints in your lobby.
- The person whose eyes won't dilate or constrict.
- Sutures.
- Missing muscles on one side of the neck.
- Acting clueless in the face of a major health issue. The classic example is a gentleman who had spent five years on a special issuance for a prior issue and then acted baffled (and flew for six months) when the issue came back again. Even though he had been legally warned that he couldn't fly if it returned, he ignored that directive and did it anyway.
- No…not really.
- "So, doc, what all is on the exam?"
- "We didn't do this last time." (Yeah, we did.)
- Folks who continuously remind you that they've referred people to you. Now, this might be pity—perhaps they simply gazed around your office. But keep your eyes open. Coercion begins with flattery.
- New pilots who repeatedly name-drop other pilots you may know or who referred them to you. Even better, those who mention that they know a lot of other pilots and would be happy to refer them to you. This may again just be a sign of a good person being nice, but turn on the radar set just in case a bogey tries to penetrate.
- People who try to frame the situation they are in—they're six minutes into the discussion, and you have yet to hear the medical condition you'll be helping them with. Any time a patient attempts to limit or frame the discussion, you'd better be wary.
- Not knowing the names of your daily medications is a huge medical red flag.
- Not knowing why you take your daily medications.
- Preening about your former competency. I remember one gentleman who went out of his way to repeatedly tell that he had been a highly skilled, top-level engineer for years. I woke up after a while, deferred his exam, and calmly let him know that I was

far more concerned about his present lack of judgment in trying to hide several medical issues from a physician who felt every bit as competent as he was once upon a distant time.
- Another gentleman spent a lot of time talking about how he was just as healthy today as he was in the past, but when I put him through his vision testing, he subtly changed to, "Not bad for a seventy-four-year-old." When he exhibited major limitations in his back and extremities examination, he became less subtle: "Well, I am seventy-four years old; what do you expect?" Remember: The airplane has no idea or concern what age you are; it only demands your full competency during the most trying situations.
- Sometimes a pilot may remember a medication, but if they suddenly remember a couple of new ones while you are going over their history, that is something to keep a careful eye on.
- A common red flag is the pilot who gets on the table and says, "I didn't know how to put this on the form, but…" Yeah, thanks. You just made everyone's day a little tougher by your intentional subterfuge. And you turned my radar set to high.

My son will attest that I sometimes just get a little crabby about the silliest stuff, although my sense of humor is getting better at turning the crabbiness into a joke on myself. But there was one day before I had learned that vital skill of self-deprecation, when a guy walked in with no appointment. I confronted him with, "What are you doing here? You know you need to make an appointment!" I quickly discovered he was just bringing in some magazines for my lobby. *Oops.*

Or in LateLiarEnglish,

> Me: I can be a jerk.
> Him: Yeah, but you're our jerk.

16

What Brings You to My Business Today, Doc?

or, Never Park Your Ice Cream Truck in My Lobby

Oh, the stories I have...

The pickle guy: A person new to our practice walked into the office and slammed five plastic containers of pickles onto the intake desk. They went flying, sending pickle juice all over the office. He did apologize, but it was a bit late. Dr. Jekyll had left the building seconds before in a mist of vinegar and cucumber seeds.

▲ ▲ ▲

Mangosteen: A certain pilot's wife took up an hour of the office staff's time, marketing her product. Multilevel marketing used to happen a lot more, but I have figured out the proper grip-and-throw technique for extricating these folks. I also asked for their business license and for rent money and threatened them with eviction. After all, it was my office space they were trying to sublet.

Neon drink: Tastes like *crap*! Don't market energy drinks to a doctor who still has taste buds and who was hospitalized as a child for drinking ethylene glycol...especially if your product tastes like ethylene glycol.

Wait Your Turn: Lady walked in, and I was busy. I told her the usual—"We do exams only by appointment. We are booked up right now, but if you call us in a little bit, we'll get you done." Of course that simply wasn't good enough, but I told her we have a lot of people here, and she will have to wait her turn.

She walked directly outside and immediately called me to make an appointment, literally three seconds after I told her to call us in a little bit. Then she kept calling when I didn't answer. On the sixth call, I answered and she started off *muy rapido, cuando yo solamente habla despacio.* I already knew she spoke perfect English, so I told her, "Look, call me back in about three hours. I am busy."

Instead, she walked back into the busy office and demanded information. At that moment, she was asked to leave. When she refused, I pulled out my phone and said, "I am calling 911 to have you arrested for trespassing. If you don't leave now—"

She began describing my full evolutionary lineage in graphic detail, pausing only to affect a head wave or a finger waggle. The 911 operator came on speakerphone.

I said, "I am a doctor. I have asked this person repeatedly to leave, but she simply won't. She is interrupting my ability to do my job in certifying immigrants such as herself to come into this country. I am thinking we need to consider Baker Acting her or at least removing her to a deportation center, because she clearly isn't all here. If she were, she'd recognize the position she is putting herself in…Oh wait. She walked out, ma'am. I think that got through to her. Sorry to waste your time."

I have no idea if she was selling things or trying to set up an appointment, but the attitude is identical. Forget that it's your office, doc, this is my agenda and all must bow to my presence.

▲ ▲ ▲

It's always important to be aware that you are at *my* business receiving *my* wares. Unless you have a business license with my address on it, it probably isn't a good idea to come into my office to try to sell me your agenda. Especially if you are supposed to be there for a flight physical but really want to push your latest multilevel marketing find. Be prepared—I may ask you for rent.

17

Dealing with the Feds

or, How I Hope Semmelweis Isn't Applauding Me at the Moment

THIS CHAPTER NEEDS a preface, because if you simply read it without understanding that it contains anecdotes of *rare events* and not *common ones*, you might think I hold the Aerospace Medical Certification Division (AMCD) in low regard. This is not the case. These people have a very difficult and unenviable job, and with constant influx/efflux of personnel at the FAA management levels above them, many times they are caught up in situations not of their making. The bad decisions surrounding the very good CACI worksheets may have been one of those times. But, again, if it seems I am biting the hand that feeds me, I truly am only nibbling without breaking the skin. When I break the skin, I'll have the condiments ready.

I have never laughed harder at a poor decision than when the CACI worksheets came into being. They were a great idea, but an utterly silly melodrama tainted their first six months of origination. The CACI worksheets began as a chance to allow AMEs greater latitude in decision-making for some common issues such as hypertension and hypothyroidism. They also provided latitude on uncommon issues such as cases of bladder and testicular cancer, which I see once every four years or so on average in my very busy aviation medicine practice.

Soon after the worksheets were initiated, we were sent surveys via the messaging system that we were required to complete before we could log into our own pilot's files. Essentially, we were locked out of our own practice until we answered these nonsensical survey questions. The most comical questions were about how comfortable we were with the new protocols and whether these protocols would change our approach to patients with bladder cancer or testicular cancer or hypertension. Of course, if you treat something daily, you quickly memorize a protocol to use; thus, there is no real change except during the initial learning curve and then you get comfortable with the change. The changes were minor to begin with for the common items, and if you rarely or never see a condition such as bladder or renal cancer in a pilot, it doesn't matter if there is a new protocol—you're still going to handle that situation the same way you would any other uncommon issue. You'll look up what to do and follow the guidelines.

Hell, three quarters of flight doctors have likely not had a pilot with bladder cancer in the past ten years. Thus, their comfort level is equal no matter what change is made; they are simply going to go look up what they are to do.

Let's take bladder cancer for example. The average age at diagnosis is seventy-three. That eliminates all but about thirty thousand pilots, if that many. The risk of occurrence in their lives is one in twenty-six, so of those affected, I'd estimate that probably twelve hundred will get bladder cancer.

Of those who do, one in five will be very sick and likely not come to get a medical because they will be grossly ill; another one in five will decide not to fly because they are undergoing treatment. What pushes them out of the cockpit is a culmination of other medical issues combined with the bladder cancer.

So we are talking about a very small number of pilots who will show up with bladder cancer, spread out among three thousand flight doctors. My approach is going to be the exact same as my approach is with lupus.

I am totally comfortable with handling both, and I will look up what I am supposed to do.

What is there to feel uncomfortable about? It is only going to happen about one time every three years—less than that if they read this book, because they are going to let me know well in advance of their exam, and we are going to handle it early and get it over with.

About half of certified flight doctors do fifty exams or fewer per year; these AMEs are probably never going to have more than a single pilot with bladder cancer in their career.

Anyway, I was still chuckling about the survey when a few weeks later we got an e-mail stating that we would now have to use specific wording when handling these protocols. In other words, we couldn't say "HTN controlled" and instead we had to type "CACI qualified hypertension." This was funny since they were supposed to be freeing us to have more autonomy, but they handcuffed us from using normal communication instead.

Whoever came up with the idea may simply have never once typed HTN instead of hypertension. If so, I do feel pity. If you needed to search something fast and had bothered to involve the flight doctors, then CACI HTN or CACI DEFER HTN would make a heck of a lot more sense, but evidently having office staff completely switch their forty years of "HTN" and "MET" to "hypertension" and "qualified" was a very important issue to someone.

I've heard rumors regarding why this exact wording was so important, but I'm a little wary of rumors. For years, FAA personnel told me the reason we were using an 1864 post—Civil War modem instead of a more modern system of ECG transmission was because the signal quality couldn't be equaled by PDF files.

After witnessing ten years of this, an e-mail arrives stating that, due to the poor quality of modem transmitted ECGs, we would instead begin submitting the much higher quality ECGs...by computer via PDF file.

Thus, rumors from back channels aren't always to be trusted. After all, I knew the whole time that "modem signal quality" was a myth. Sometimes it would be simpler and saner to just say, "I don't know." But that seems to be an unnatural response for humans.

This whole CACI wording nonsense was silly, especially if they were doing it solely for being able to do a word search (according to one rumor). After all, you are only going to end up with a few hundred bladder cancers in the entire FAA database, so typing "CACI met bladder cancer" won't save that much time from simply typing "Bladder Ca." It is pretty comical that you'd impair three thousand flight doctors and their staff solely for the rare case when you are studying incidence and protocols on a rarely occurring issue.

The more common items such as hypothyroidism or hypertension are already searchable. Did they mark "yes" to the hypertension box? Did they input "thyroid" or "Synthroid" or "levothyroxine"? Then you'll quickly accomplish a data count on those patients as well.

Half of AMEs are older and have a well-established office staff. The FAA set itself up to fail because people don't like changes, especially people who have been sitting at a desk doing things the same way for sixty years.

And stir up a hornet's nest it did. For me, it was like watching *The Three Stooges*, because I'd been to enough FAA meetings to know that our geriatric AMEs were going to be stirred up. Hell, it's the most redeeming quality of being forced to go to an in-person meeting in an era of modern Internet connectivity. The scourges of the condominium were turning their attention to AMCD, as a manner of speaking.

For the next three months, I literally was rolling laughing as reminder after reminder issued themselves from the FAA: "The CACI phrasing must be absolutely word for word." The height of the fun was when the federal air surgeon's letter mentioned that, after several months, they still had only a 25 percent accuracy rate. That ruined all the fun for me, since I had made a bet with myself that their accuracy rate wouldn't have topped 5 percent, because every single AME affected would have realized that none of the other AMEs were going to go along with this and thus they were all having a wildcat strike asked as ignorance.

Of course, I had been using the exact phrasing, word for word, from the get-go. Watching that totally flawed process work itself into a well-rutted, insipidly broken maturation when it could have been done with ease and professionalism was the source of a lot of mirth. I still can't believe that AMCD was able to get accuracy up to 25 percent so quickly. I would have bet they would never have reached 20 percent, ever. Apparently, cajoling repeatedly for six months did pay off, even if the FAA didn't understand what a marvelous result the cajoling had produced. They were looking victory in the face and declaring a defeat.

I work hard to create an attitude of collegiality when talking to the folks in Oklahoma City, where the main medical staff of the FAA work. The process of calling them involves first speaking to a nongovernment employee who then can route you to the doctors if you need further assistance.

At one time, there was a non-FAA employee who would routinely refuse to allow me to talk to the physicians there, because evidently in her mind, a verbal authorization was an assault on everything she held dear. I would have to call two or three times and hang up every time I heard her voice, but eventually, I would get someone different, and right to the doc I'd be sent. Apparently, enough complaints were eventually lodged against this person that AMCD cleaned up the matter.

Over the years, when I've had problems or questions, I've done my absolute best not to violate the AME guide (our protocol bible of four hundred or so pages and growing). Instead, diligently, I first research all the Federal Air Surgeons Bulletins in the archives. Then, if I am still not clear, I move on to the phone call. Often, in the past, I could save AMCD personnel an awful lot of time by gathering all the information that I knew they would need on a new student pilot and then call AMCD, give the doctor the information over the phone, and then fax or mail the hard copies.

This verbal authorization process worked very well on two fronts. One, it ensured that the pilot was handled promptly and didn't join a growing pile of work to be done. Two, I used it as a powerful tool to eradicate myths that student pilots hear from their fellows about how mean and evil AMCD can be. In addition, it seemed to me that helping a student pilot realize that AMCD is a helpful entity out to address their issues, is simply good marketing and good business. First impressions.

For me, quickly certifying a pilot is a way to contravene misinformation while providing both the pilot and AMCD direct benefit. However, collegiality isn't always a two-way street, and it has led to some good comedy, as well as some eye-opening rethinking of what the AMCD is really all about.

Perhaps the best line I have ever heard to describe the doctor group at AMCD is, "John, we have ten doctors and eleven opinions." And seriously, that concept is as good as any to explain the occasional weird things that occur. It especially comes into play whenever there is a change in personnel at AMCD. An AME does well to realize that what you did yesterday may change tomorrow based solely on the comfort level of the person at the other end of the line. Thus, plan your conversations to establish trust and ease any possible concerns the folks on the other end of the line may have about the particular case you are discussing.

▲ ▲ ▲

One day, I had a relatively easy phone call to make regarding a pilot with hypertension. Now, in the AME guide, hypertension isn't an issue that requires a special issuance, and I had been doing these exams for ten years. It had never been called a special issuance by anyone ever in my recollection. So, suddenly in the middle of the phone call, I found myself in a heated exchange with an FAA doctor who was insisting that hypertension is a special-issuance condition, and I was caught so off guard that I fell into my own emotions and become inappropriately heated as well. I had flown into IFR conditions without even realizing there was a cloud in the sky.

Finally, after a lot of silly back-and-forth that wasn't productive at all, I figured out (or it was explained to me) that there are special issuances and there are special issuances (unwritten, in the AME guide). In other words, after ten years of being an AME, I had discovered that there were two separate set of guidelines that had two different sets of definitions… or something, because I had no access to any of this backroom, hidden bible.

Now, I am not being paranoid—this was actually what I was told and what was later confirmed via careful observation and repeated confirmation, both by regional flight surgeons and by AMCD physicians. This should raise a few eyebrows. And, I am not clairvoyant, but I suspect the presence of two separate sets of definitions and guidelines can be traced back to another issue AMCD has. AMCD and the federal air surgeon branch of the DOT often lack the most basic common sense when it comes to intelligence gathering and decision-making.

That said, they do create surveys…but their surveys ask questions that *they* think are important. And that is an inherently flawed setup. Also, they buffer the answers. Out of three thousand plus flight doctors, half of them do less than one FAA medical exam per week. You are surveying people who clearly don't handle the volume needed to give you well-qualified, experienced, reasonable comments based upon an adequate sample size of pilots.

When you use a survey where half of the surveyed persons aren't that vested in the whole process, you water down the comments of real value by spacing them out among a disproportionately larger set of responses that might as well come from a Baskin Robbins employee. If a flight doctor isn't doing three or four medicals per week at the very minimum, I don't think they are going to feel the real impact of changes to the system, such as a person doing ten or twelve exams a week will feel. Nor do I think they will have thought out their solutions fully before they institute changes that impact the people they've put at the frontline and entrusted to carry out an important duty.

Until you ask first and solve problems second, you will just be chasing your tail. Your thinking that you know the answers to my problems is a poor substitute to listening to me talk about what my problems are in the first place.

A practical example of this is the sleep apnea fiasco, wherein scientifically the FAA was so totally correct, and yet from an implementation standpoint, the FAA created its own self-consuming firestorm and maybe pushed the GA community further toward the Pilot's Bill of Rights 2 nonsense.

And there lies the issue. The FAA quite often makes decisions, places policies into place, and never seems to adequately vet their new ideas with the people in the field who are doing the real hard work—the flight doctors. At times, the FAA even does things that are almost the reverse of what is in their own best interests. I will get back to the sleep apnea fiasco later, as it deserves its own chapter, but first, let me get back to the new student pilots to illustrate my point in the last sentence. AMCD sometimes does things that conflict with their own best interests.

▲ ▲ ▲

One day, I had a new pilot come into my office with a previous medical condition that required me to defer the decision-making to AMCD. I had the pilot gather up all the material he needed, then counseled and consoled him, assuring him that this was not a big deal. After all, I had for years been able to call the FAA at AMCD and verbally get authority to issue. So I called the FAA, and the nongovernment employee who answered their phone told me in no uncertain terms that I was not going to be able to talk to a doctor about this issue for two reasons. First, it was a Tuesday and they were no longer taking phone calls on Tuesday, and second, they would no longer discuss medical issues on student pilots. The AME had to send the deferral in and the student pilot could just wait the six weeks or more for the AMCD to decide what they were going to do with the case. I was beyond shocked, since this nongovernmental employee had refused to even let me confer with an FAA employee to confirm this matter. I called the Southern Region. Sure enough, that was the new policy and rather than discuss, ask for input, or even e-mail via the online mandatory messaging center that we often must read prior to logging into the system—they had instead allowed nongovernment employees to be the fall people. These employees had to field thousands of calls from irate AMEs (not me, I found it comical), who now had to explain to thousands of student pilots that their flight instructors were right when they called the AMCD all kinds of names.

The bad policy of that whole situation was beyond explanation, particularly when this online messaging center was used regularly for the most esoteric of news, including one e-mail all of us doctors received that touted how successful the new system was...but which ironically then seemed to cause the new system to crash.

In fairness, the new system—now that it's debugged—is outstanding. But not to escape from the salient issue, it was patently bad decision-making to hide behind nongovernment contractors. There was already a messaging system in place, debugged for months, that would have saved AMCD dozens and dozens of phone calls and not cost AMEs time, energy, and bad outcomes with pilots who were new to aviation and were experiencing their first impressions of AMCD's decision-making process while feeling lied to by their AME.

It did, indeed, make AMEs look like liars to the student pilots whom they had told they would be able to help and then couldn't. And it made AMCD seem punitive to the student pilots. Not having time to plan and inform the flight schools of these changes so that we could all implement policy changes prior to the AMCD policy change also gave the flight schools a negative opinion of the situation. All of this was totally avoidable and created unneeded animosity and rumor about AMCD and its decision-making processes.

But the all-time great comedic moment was the day I was trying my best to help a pilot, make the system work, ensure the pilot was vetted, and use the tools given to me.

▲ ▲ ▲

A local AME had retired, and I was the recipient of a lot of the pilots who had visited him for years. Many were on hypertension medication, and he had been doing a good job of ensuring that they were reporting this and that their doctors were providing him with feedback. In fact, his partner often acted as a primary care doctor for many of his patients, including the pilot who was in my office that day.

Now, most pilots, laypersons, sod tillers, and Amish would assume that if you have a huge online database medical record-keeping system, that when you go to an AME, they can see all of your past aviation exam information. That would be incorrect. The good news is that there are personnel in AMCD working on this issue. Because obviously, if I have a pilot who has been on the same hypertension medication for fifteen years and has thirty exams showing good BP control, then that is about the best possible evidence of good hypertension control that an AME will ever get in their lifetime. After all, thirty times someone checked his BP, and thirty times it met the FAA standard—plus any other reports from his treating doctor would also have been included into the database. In addition to that, the pilot had no real vested interest in lying, since they had already been reporting BP and already reporting they take medication. A good historian can see if the pilot is giving off any red flags as well.

That said, the FAA policy on hypertension is germane to this story. The policy states that the pilot must provide the AME yearly status reports from the pilot's treating physician *or* (the most important *or*), if the AME can otherwise determine that the pilot has been stable on medication for at least seven days, then the AME can certify the pilot. This is really important, because the FAA designed this specifically to free up the AME to be more autonomous in using their judgment to determine whether the pilot's BP is well controlled.

The FAA didn't specify any parameters whatsoever concerning what constitutes a *proper* versus *improper* AME decision. It leaves the decision 100 percent up to the AME. It makes the AME the game designer of the game called "is this pilot's BP controlled for more than seven days." In fact, in a recent meeting with eighty AME physicians, the FAA speaker stated clearly that they had designed the CACI system to allow the AME to be the decision-maker and that they would trust our judgment on these medical issues.

Now, of course, the third set of rules the FAA has can always be used—"You are outta here." This rule exists as guard against an AME whose idea of game design is simply inane or dishonest. Thus, if the FAA thinks an AME is a bad actor, they can send that person right out the door. And rightfully so.

In my way of thinking then, if the pilot gives me a good history, shows no signs of obfuscation, presents no red flags, and has been going for years to a flight physician I have had the chance to observe and who has been very good in dealing with hypertension, then that by itself could be a proper determination in some AMEs minds.

But to me, as my own personal FAA-appointed game designer, I felt more comfortable calling the FAA to obtain the information about his past thirty visits, which the FAA was actively working on making available to me anyway as numerous doctors, including one earlier that very day, had told me was occurring. So out came the cell phone, and I called the FAA on speed dial.

OK, enough boring stuff. Now for the comedy.

"Hey, this is doctor Shewmaker. Can you tell me what BP medication and dosage Pilot Bob was on during his past two visits?"

"Sure. Looks like his last physician report was last year and he was on medication X." (This is the same thing he was on today.)

"Great, what about six months ago?"

"Oh, he didn't do a doctor report six months ago."

"I know. What medications did he report on his flight exam six months ago?"

"Oh...you'll need to get a new physician report; it's been a year."

"Was he on the same medication and dosage six months ago?"

"Yes, but he needs a new physician report."

OK, let's pause here. At this point, an astute physician would have realized they were talking to the gateway personnel and not the decision-makers and said, "You are so right!" and hung up the phone and issued the medical to the pilot.

But me, astute? I wasn't feeling it. Instead, I got myself caught trying to help this poor, clearly untrained person by trying to be friendly and educate her.

So I said, "Actually, the new CACI protocol allows the physician to issue if they can otherwise determine that the BP is well controlled." After all, I had no idea if this person got hired a day ago and of what kind of training she had undergone. Let me help her out, and she'll appreciate my assistance. Uh, not so much.

From there it was, "No, you need a report."

"But I really don't..."

And so on for a few silly cycles of totally unnecessary drivel back and forth, until my mind was drawn to the thoughts of Diet Coke, and I hung up laughing to myself about how poorly my attempt at covering all the bases and making sure this pilot was on the up and up had gone. But I did feel comfortable knowing this pilot had been well controlled for at least two separate visits in the past year and was well controlled on his visit to me as well. So, PRINT CERTIFICATE, pilot CACI qualified hypertension. Word for word. Exactly. I had met my definition of "AME can otherwise determine..."

Of course, I explained to the pilot that if they ever get the online system fixed to allow us to see old exams from other flight doctors, this silliness wouldn't happen. He politely didn't say that they could also fix it by getting AMEs astute enough not to waste time on the non decision maker's misconceptions of a clearly spelled-out-in-English verbatim guideline. So this guy clearly met my FAA appointed determination that he was in good control for blood pressure, and off he went with a medical.

Ten minutes later, I got a phone call from an AMCD doctor who attempted to play "I am the cougar on this range, can't you smell that pee on the trees?" I wasn't in the mood because I was laughing too hard. He was probably a bit caught off guard when I cut him off midsentence.

He started off with, "We don't appreciate it when doctors try to game the system—" He didn't get much further, however, because he listened to me explain in detail how offensive it was to be accused of gaming the system when the CACI protocols gave me the right to otherwise determine. Furthermore, it was hardly gaming the system if I was calling them on my time to get information in order to make a good decision.

Hell, if I were going to game the system, calling them up to get old information would be the absolutely last thing I would do. I am a business owner, and wasting time on phone calls isn't a good "gaming the system" concept if I were a "gaming the system" sort of person. Patently, that was not a well thought out claim by the other party, but we often don't think, we just react. And that is what seemed to be happening on the other end of the line. This phone call to me was a knee-jerk reaction. Understandable—we all knee-jerk on occasion, but why did this knee jerk occur, specifically?

The accusation was logically untenable. It was impossible for me to game the system since AMCD had put me in charge of designing the rules of the game. The game is called "AME can otherwise determine"... so, I was the game designer. In essence, the person who told me that it was my decision to make was telling me that I was gaming myself by deciding how I was going to design to rules of the game I had been placed in charge of designing.

When I clearly explained to him that if I just had access to the pilot's past thirty visits demonstrating controlled BP while on the same medication, that that would convince the most skeptical person of the pilot having excellent blood pressure control, he was able to get in his punchline: "Oh, I know. We are working on that."

So, in essence, he told me they were working on a system to allow me to do what I was already doing, except I wouldn't have to call them at all to get the information that they were working on making more available to me...and I am getting a headache typing this. Apparently, I was gaming the system by doing exactly what they were working on doing for me? ¡Ay caramba!

Naturally, I left that phone call and began a long, tearful process of heaving, laughing, and rolling on the floor until I began considering why a doctor would call me, begin by demeaning me, and never apparently assume that I had anything but good intentions. Of course, all I had were the purest of good intentions, because in both of the two phone calls, I had been trying to help them and to make the system work smoothly.

It had one plausible explanation that I placed onto the decision tray of Occam's Razor and which to me makes the most sense. They must field so many calls from doctors who truly do try to game the system that this poor fellow assumed I was a salmon like all the other salmon. I am a perch. Now a smart doctor who *was* trying to game the system would likely not go out of the way to call AMCD. But perhaps on the occasion that they did call, their words and statements might show a casual approach or a lack of basic aviation medicine knowledge that could cause AMCD over time to develop a concern about their average flight doctor in the field.

A careful reflection then would also be to ask if is there a damaged relationship between AMCD and some of the less vested flight doctors. These anecdotes do tend to shade that nuance. And if that is the case—that AMCD has a healthy distrust of some AMEs based upon the typical phone calls that AMCD fields, and that causes them to overreact to a benign phone call such as my own—then AMCD has a large problem on its hands. You can't run a system if you have developed a nagging suspicion about the underlying motivations of your field personnel. And if your nagging suspicions are actually correct, then you have not only a large problem on your hands, you have a problem that greatly endangers the general public. For if there are large numbers of AMEs who truly are gaming the system or making phone calls that would make the AMCD folks suspect them, then a lot of sick pilots could very well be slipping through the cracks. It's something to ponder.

▲ ▲ ▲

Another funny incident was the incandescent light bulb issue. I had been saving that one for darker day, but one day, the FAA called my hand on it. I got a call stating that I wasn't putting in the uncorrected vision on my forms for pilots who wore glasses. Well, being fairly well versed in this topic, I knew that in 2008 they had changed the policy to allow us to leave off this completely unneeded data, since if the person required glasses, it was wholly irrelevant how illegally blind they were when they illegally flew without their legally required glasses. But it did take a while to find evidence, and so when I finally found the federal air surgeon's letters to the editor in 2008 or 2009 stating that it was no longer necessary to put down uncorrected values or to make pilot remove contact lenses, I sent that up the chain.

Never to yet hear back, by the way, on the definitive ruling, but as we were chuckling at this one, I brought something else up to one of the FAA physicians. Three years ago, the US government phased out 100-watt incandescent bulbs, yet the FAA required us to all have 100-watt incandescent bulbs above our eye charts.

A flurry of e-mails began to fly, so you can blame me for some of the increased national debt as this flurry doubtless took hours of needed work away from already overworked FAA personnel. Not really sure yet how that will all work out. But, I'll leave the light on for them.

Meanwhile, I have since attended an FAA conference where an FAA doctor stated clearly during his talk that you did not need to remove contact lenses when checking vision on pilots. So, right hand, let me introduce you to left hand. These things are simply a byproduct of size. Large organizations often have small communications issues wherein different groups inadvertently use different information. It happens.

Expect multiple small errors within large organizations in flux.

And now let us move on to the sleep apnea fiasco. Here, poor planning caused the FAA to paint itself into a corner that it doesn't yet seem to realize it is in.

18

Rip Van Winkle

or, How Bad Decisions Are Like Freeze-Dried Dandelion Seeds

SLEEP APNEA IS a very big issue. It is especially common in very large people and is associated with a host of other serious medical issues. Unarguably, people die on the highways when they are tired. There are plenty of data regarding the effect of fatigue on drivers.

So when the FAA published that sleep apnea is almost ubiquitous in people over a neck size of seventeen and a BMI of forty, they in effect placed a real policy change into the hands of all AMEs who were honest and paying attention. Why? Because if I strongly suspect that a patient has sleep apnea or any other medical condition, I have an obligation at that moment to defer that person until my suspicion of sleep apnea is proven unfounded. And since there are only about a thousand pilots in the United States within that criteria, then it was only going to be about one pilot affected for every three flight doctors. This really could have been handled with as little fanfare as possible and without any real change in overall policy.

For example, one scenario would be that AMCD calls the AME and tells him, "Hey, Bob has a BMI of forty and neck size of seventeen. Our data show he is likely to have sleep apnea." At that point, AMCD has painted Bob and the AME into a corner. In fact, they could have done it so quietly and so cleverly that the AME could have been the real driver of the conversation and no policy change was ever needed.

The FAA could simply have repeatedly put articles discussing how often apnea is missed into the Federal Air Surgeons Bulletin, while repeatedly citing the statistics that a BMI of forty and a neck size of seventeen is a virtual guarantee on sleep apnea.

This pressure would have been felt downstream solely by the AME, not the pilot, not the AOPA, and not the Congress with its geriatric pilot and his meddling vendettas. And if the pressure subtly placed on the AME wasn't felt to the satisfaction of AMCD, then a phone call by a regional flight surgeon to discuss a particular case would have had the overall necessary outcome.

This was about defining standard of care, which doesn't require federal involvement beyond very craftily repeating over and over, whispering into the ear of the AMEs that BMI forty/neck size seventeen equals a virtually guaranteed apnea. After all, the AME can ignore AMCD, but he likely won't if he is repeatedly hearing that his patient is guaranteed to have apnea. No, the AME is going to warn Bob early to go get a sleep study (which is the smart thing to do), while telling Bob it's his idea because of some studies he'd just seen. The AME is going to tell Bob he is worried about him and his health. (Be the hero; save the guy's life; take all the credit.) Either that or the AME will wait until Bob comes in and be silly, deferring Bob, blaming AMCD, and thus creating a combative situation wherein a pilot blames the FAA. But that won't trickle out to the EAA or the AOPA either. Every deferred pilot is a potential rumor spreader already, so the impact would have been diluted.

Couple this with a smart AMCD phone call that discusses options (code talk for "spells out the benefit to the AME of calling Bob and being the hero, not the deferring agent"), and we would have that policy in place and at the most only one in every five flight doctors would even know about it. Further, most of those flight doctors who were called will think it is only that one guy they happen to have in their practice and not even dwell on the fact that the FAA rarely calls. An even subtler approach would be the "oh, by the way" call, a technique that I use all the time. AMCD could call up the AME and mention some other issues of importance, and in passing drop strong hints about that one guy who was there six months ago who is a guaranteed lock to have sleep apnea.

"Hey, if the guy does have sleep apnea, you could do him a favor by getting him checked now. Our data say he is a virtual lock; so does the literature. But if you get his sleep apnea treated well before his exam comes due next year, we can have him on a special issuance before that time comes, and he won't lose a single day of flying. You can be the hero, here."

It really could have been that easy. A side benefit of focusing on this method of addressing the most probable affected pilots is that the AME would become educated more fully on looking at the other signs of sleep apnea, such as jaw shape, tongue, and oropharynx appearance. Additionally, AMEs would have increased screening and discussion with these pilots about the need to think about weight control and possible sleep apnea testing. Sometimes subtly striking a facet at a time results in a much better gemstone than crushing it with a compacter.

Tightening of the sleep apnea standards could then have happened stepwise, as more and more AMEs were prodded about a case or two. It didn't need much pressure; it just needed focused pressure at the right point. Besides, the FAA policy had already stated that if an AME thinks that a patient has an illness, the AME has an obligation to explore. That was always the case.

Thus, the forty BMI/seventeen neck pilot would have failed the medical exam if they had gone to a flight doctor well trained in the statistics of sleep apnea prior to the FAA stepping in and trying to institute a new policy.

In other words, before the new sleep apnea policy began its tortured comedic entrance, doctors who thought patients had sleep apnea were already under the obligation to further examine this by sending them out to a sleep specialist. It's the same as if you looked at a person with a nasal polyp and were obligated to get that pilot an ENT evaluation. Sleep apnea was already a disease requiring a special issuance.

Instead, the FAA took an opposite approach and telegraphed a wide set of sweeping changes that were about to occur—without clearly elucidating them—to a group associated with more bad rumors than a knitting circle in winter in a small farming community. I have no doubt this was with all the best intentions.

The policy would have pandered to sleep study specialists who would have preyed on naïve patients and billed them for both a home and an office sleep study, when they already knew they would fail the home study. The FAA's own data predicted that the home study would almost always result in a failure, thus it was useless to even do one. In fact, during a recent talk to flight doctors, an FAA lecturer who was a sleep study specialist put it succinctly: "Home sleep studies suck." That is a verbatim quote from a speech on January 30, 2016, given to over seventy flight doctors.

This started a firestorm of controversy from every single alphabet soup in the aviation community. The cries of foul (or fowl, because some pilots can't spell all that well) came to be heard on the floors of Congress, and so much pressure came down, led by the octogenarian pilot who once missed a huge X on a runway, that a new meeting was held and every one was invited to participate in a teleconference.

The entire discussion of fatigue and aircraft accidents is irrelevant since the discussion is fatigue. Thus, any kind of accident anywhere in any form of transportation is relevant.

Once causality is established, the vehicle isn't important unless it knows what kind of vehicle it is—and none of them do. And so after a lot of thought, I finally realized the stratagem needed to accomplish my goal was to gently point out some issues that didn't seem to have been raised. The strategy became to ask a two-part question. I would ask it calmly, and I would try to do so during the most heated part of the debate.

Set the trap with question one.

Spring the trap with question two.

I wanted to ask a cutting question that would put the person into a box wherein "no," "I don't know," or "yes" would equally trap that person by one of three secondary questions attacking the answer the person gave. However, I wanted it to be hidden in the invective of a large group, so that only I remembered who asked it.

So the teleconference started, and about a half an hour in, I keyed in my question. A soft-spoken moderator (which was perfect, because my voice was too deep for the strategy to work to perfection) read it. The question went to the federal air surgeon: "Since a large majority of these morbidly obese patients are in the third-class medical certificate group, do you foresee a possibility that a great many of them may simply ignore the FAA's concern and give up their medical and go light sport?"

Now, that is a trap.

The right answer is yes, because it is the correct answer. If he says yes, however, the alphabet people are going to say that the new sleep apnea policy was obviously flawed. (And it was, solely because this would have happened—most of the affected pilots would have likely just gone light sport and flown with untreated sleep apnea.) As sick as it sounds, many pilots care far more about their ability to have a hobby than they do about their personal health, which would enable them to pursue their hobby for a longer period of their lives.

I planned that if he said no, then he'd get a really good second question proving this happens regularly. If he said "I don't know," then he would be trapped into admitting he doesn't have the data to make a change…and the alphabet people would temporarily rejoice until I spring the second question to close the trap on everyone.

Well, the federal air surgeon did me one better. He said, "Well, I would be very disappointed in them if they did that."

What the air surgeon had just said was that he would be disappointed in a group of people making a decision to go into a class less restrictive upon them—a class the FAA itself had created specifically to allow less restriction to exist for these pilots!

What he seemed not to grasp was that these pilots chose to fly in that class for one reason only—they don't care about your, my, or the federal air surgeon's emotions. They don't want our input about their health. These pilots don't give one rat's ass about your, mine or the FAA's levels of disappointment—that's their whole point in lobbying to get you the hell out of their lives in the first place. That is the whole point of the LSA class, from a pilot's point of view.

For many pilots, the response to his disappointment would likely be a protracted yawn. Unfortunate? Yes. Fact? Absolutely.

Part two of the question came five minutes later. "Given that many pilots have already foregone the third-class medical and gone LSA for issues such as Alzheimer's, Parkinson's, metastatic cancers, heart disease, COPD, and so on, which is actually more dangerous to the public? The pilots who have sleep apnea or the LSA class itself?"

And the air surgeon walked right back in, chewed on the bait, watched the door swing shut, and didn't even realize he was in a trap. "Well, I don't know if that is correct about these pilots going LSA, and again, I would be very disappointed in them."

Again, this overlooks the salient point that these pilots simply aren't going to care about the federal air surgeon's disappointment. It is nowhere near their radar. It also overlooks the fact that LSA is exactly about sick pilots giving up medicals and flying dangerously.

There was a lot of invective in that teleconference, but I do know they canceled the policy the very next day, and came up with a new, equally flawed, and equally comical policy with its own set of unique silliness about a year later.

So what policy did the FAA finally come up with?

Well, they decided sleep apnea was so important that they added one whole page to the four pages of the FAA medical exam website and promptly gutted the entire screening of sleep apnea, consequently placing the AME into a trap and themselves into a far bigger one, without them seeming to grasp it.

The new, totally flawed system is far less restrictive on pilots, and has far less chance of being truly effective.

It divides pilots into six categories, including a category to grandfather in (without penalty) any pilot who has been lying to them for years. The main category that defeats the entire process is category five:

This category is for people that the AME considers "At risk for OSA. AASM sleep apnea assessment required. Reports to follow."

So, what are these assessments? First, the pilot is given the certificate. Then the pilot is allowed to go to their own doctor, and if that doctor writes a letter clearing them, they need no sleep study. Far less onerous but far more dangerous, because it takes almost nothing for pilots to find a doctor stupid enough to ignore reality and write a nonsensical clearing letter.

These doctors already are a penny a dozen, and the pilots know that.

Secondly, if the AME uses the FAA's own position—that a person with a BMI of forty and a neck size of seventeen is virtually a guaranteed sleep apnea patient—the AME and the FAA are essentially closing their eyes to the facts as they exist medically and allowing a non-FAA trained doctor who may be the pilot's next door neighbor to simply scrawl on a report that the pilot isn't apneic. And as hard as it might be for a naïve person to believe, these doctors exist en masse.

You have zero idea of the private physician's basic knowledge on a specific disease, yet you are asking that person to certify that the pilot doesn't have a risk for that disease after you, yourself, *knowing those data*, already know that there is a massively high probability that the pilot does, in fact, have the disease.

It's a great way to claim you did your best, but in reality it is simply shaking your head gently into the sand and wriggling your tail feathers in the air.

I think it somewhat dangerous to pretend to be pro safety, while ignoring your own data and reality and pretending to create a charade of a policy, especially when you have daily reminders from non-FAA, non-AME physicians that these physicians aren't taking your requests for pilot evaluations seriously.

But the strangest part of the whole sleep apnea fiasco occurred three months after they canceled their really bad attempt to openly institute a policy they didn't need to implement.

A gentleman with a fifty-four BMI and a neck size well over twenty walked into my office. He was there for a physical; he worked for a major government organization that had been pushing the passage of a new sleep-apnea protocol for the past four months.

According to the people he works for, he had a 100 percent chance of having sleep apnea. So, he proceeded to tell me that he knows I can't pass him, but he simply needed a medical on file so that if he came back from his current medical leave, he can go back to work faster.

When I asked him what symptoms caused him to be out of work, he listed the following: eighteen months ago, he noticed fatigue, daytime somnolence, irritability, mood lability changes in his attitudes and behavior, and depressed mood. Naturally, we, the feds, and AOPA, EAA (Experimental Aircraft Association), ALPA, and anyone paying attention already knows this guy not only has sleep apnea, he's the president of the club.

So I asked him, "How did you feel when they told you that you had sleep apnea?"

"Sleep apnea? I have never been told I had that. What is it?"

Thunk, thunk, thunk.

"Sir, you couldn't be more of a poster child. You have every single symptom and every single sign of sleep apnea—from your large tongue to oropharynx ratio to your irritability and fatigue."

This gentleman was off the regression line for sleep apnea and seriously didn't even need a sleep study. You could have titrated him up on a CPAP day one, and he might have been back to work in a week.

Yet for eighteen months, he hadn't received any treatment for his highly treatable condition, partly because his primary care doctor, whom the FAA was now stating was the tip of the spear in the apnea battle, had looked right at the guy and totally missed apnea as the clear reason for his reversible symptoms. Meanwhile, the patient had possessed every single sign and symptom of sleep apnea.

I think this puts a bow on the chapter.

19

A Typical Pilot's Vision Exam

*or, **Read the Bottom Line***

Umm, let's see…F or P…maybe E, Oscar, Lima…I'm not sure…maybe G or C …umm…that could be an F, Tango, uh Papa, no Foxtrot—no, wait, P.

20

Defending Yourself for Doing Things Right

or, Do I Really Have to Pick up Another Certified Letter?

BEING A FLIGHT physician can sometimes cause other flight physicians to have their own internal war with you, while you sit back and laugh at their childishness. When I had my office in Hobe Sound, a busy flight doctor who evidently was overcharging his pilots and who didn't bother working with a pilot once they had a medical issue soon began hemorrhaging pilots to me. This was for a couple of reasons.

1. I was sending out postcards that had a pretty airplane picture and my address and mentioned that I was friendly, pilot-oriented, and fast. It also mentioned my price.
2. This seemed to be a good strategy to me, since no one likes to wait an hour to see the doctor; they want the doctor to be fast. No one wants a grouch, so I kinda pretended I wasn't. And no pilot wants to get a medical from a doctor who doesn't care at all about them being a pilot. Marketing 101.
3. The pilots were already upset with this doctor and his attitude.
4. The pilots knew the doctor's prices had become outlandish, and they felt that he was simply using them and dumping them if they became too much trouble.

So, in short, the marketing wouldn't have worked without points two, three, and four.

After a few months, pilots began telling me that I was being bad-mouthed by the doctor in question. I had to laugh, because he had just signed his articles of surrender and he hadn't even known it. After all, the pilots in his office who kept running off were being told the truth by the pilots who preceded them to my office. His slanders simply reinforced in the pilots' minds that this guy was price-gouging them.

Soon I was contacted by two flight schools farther up the coast and began doing dozens of exams on pilots from all over the world: Vietnam, Thailand, Malaysia, Iraq, Brazil…I think you are getting the point here.

These flight schools were very upset with the doctor they were using; not so much about price, but more about how inflexible and unhelpful he was with their pilots when a medical issue came up. So my practice picked up, my Spanish got better, and I even learned a couple of fascinating things about pilots who aren't primary English speakers.

Part of the FAA mandate to AMEs is that they are supposed to magically understand whether a student pilot's English skills are sufficient. This is soon changing, but at the time, the flight school would have some agitation with me when I told them I couldn't pass some of their pilots because of English proficiency issues, but we worked it out. They got to where they didn't even bat an eye when I told the Mongolian pilot that, no, I wasn't going to give him a student pilot certificate. The translator turned to him and told him what I had said, since he had no English skills at all and had shown up knowing this and bringing with him, quite politely I might add, a translator.

So about one hundred flight school students and several months later, here comes the certified letter. It basically stated that:

1. I had been accused of having three offices (which you actually could do, if you had permission, but I hadn't got permission for a third office because I didn't have a third office).
2. I had moved next to the airport and in close proximity of another flight doctor (there was no other flight doctor's office remotely close to the airport in question or either of my two offices).

3. I was passing students who couldn't speak English. (I had repeatedly not passed students specifically because they couldn't speak English and contacted the FAA to let them know, as well).

So now, here is another flight doctor shooting himself in the foot, since I immediately realized that the old flight doctor who had pissed off the flight schools was angry that he wasn't allowed to continue to be an uncaring, unapproachable jerk to the flight students. Thus, it was time for him to complain...or blow his own toes off.

So, as I am wont to do in such circumstances, I carefully pondered my approach. First I called the regional flight surgeon's office and through three or four phone calls, using each to probe carefully and solely for one clue about who was complaining, I was able to narrow it down to one flight doctor (guess who) without the regional flight surgeon's office admitting they knew what I was up to. (Hey, they are pretty smart, so for all I know they were chuckling at my subterfuge.)

Now that I was sure of who it was, I planned a maximum impact/minimum effort response. Hey, this is petty stuff, and I have a business to run. OK, I sat in the Jacuzzi and figured this out, I admit it.

1. The doctor had evidently seen a third address for me on the Internet. I had at one point received permission from the FAA to do this, but the county zoning department said I couldn't have the clinic there, so away went my deposit and my naiveté, and I told the FAA I was moving somewhere else. The Internet is like a net of bad information, though, so there were websites that listed this third nonexistent office.
2. The doctor had to have been illegally passing pilots who didn't speak any English, because the flight schools had told me I was a lot tougher on that standard. The doctor assumed I was passing these students simply because he had been passing them. This is sheer logic, because if he had real info, he'd have known that I had sent away multiple pilots and contacted the regional flight

surgeon's offices to specifically tell them about these pilots. (This was also a requirement.)
3. The doctor assumed the regional flight surgeon's offices were not going to research the proximity of offices to one another. *The Art of War* isn't that big of a book, but he obviously never read page one.

So, after a careful soaking in the hot tub, I finally called up the region.

"Hey, send me copies of the pictures, please!" I said, in a loud, begging voice (think Gilbert Godfrey).

"What pictures, Dr. Shewmaker?"

"The pictures that alleged doctor sent you of my so-called third office!"

"Uh, we don't have any pictures."

"He didn't send you a picture?"

And I know you, the reader, are smart enough to see the trap about to shut now, huh?

"OK, thanks, buh-bye," and off the phone I got just as fast as I could hang it up.

Then I mailed the letter that I had already typed up, via next-day mail, because I wanted it in their hands before they forgot I had yelled, "Hey, can you send me copies of the pictures?" Sometimes using a funny voice can help in cases like this…I was banking on it, since I do only an average Gilbert Godfrey.

The letter basically pointed out that the "third office" was currently a boat construction company office and had been for months. It also mentioned that if they rechecked the e-mails from dates x, y, and z, they would see that I had tried to change offices and told them about it, but then I also told them the move wasn't going to happen.

Then it pointed out that this complaint was clearly dishonest, since a Google map with radii on it showed I was nowhere near other flight doctors by at least three miles, and that even included the proximity of the nonexistent office to other AME offices.

And then to set the hook and reel it in, I pointed out that the only way this gentleman would have assumed I was passing non-English speakers was if he himself had been passing non-English speakers and had now lost that business through his own ineptness. This was mirrored by the fact he had made an accusation to the FAA without any visual proof of a third office, when any competent accuser with a smartphone would have been able to easily prove a third office, had it existed.

Then to gut the fish and mount it, I asked one simple question: Which is worse: a doctor with three offices, one of them without permission, or a doctor who makes up complete lies about another doctor solely for financial motives?

Now, I have never gotten their answer on that, but I did get a letter clearing me. Being not all that vindictive and knowing I am already outcompeting this rank amateur, I picked up his gutted flesh, plopped it in the deep freeze, and moved on to other things far more important than some jealous colleague. Which in my world is just about every other thing that I can think of.

▲ ▲ ▲

A side note about doing exams on foreign pilots who may be still early in their English language skills: who, what, where, why, and when questions are great ways to test comprehension. Ask an inappropriate question and watch their reaction. Here's an example:

    Me: How old are you?
    Them: Thirty-four.
    Me: Why?

For those who are still trying to learn the right words, you can almost watch their gears turning as they try to figure out if I am asking something wrong, or they are thinking something wrong. The more proficient pilot will laugh because he knows that *why* means *por que*, and understands immediately that I am joking.

▲ ▲ ▲

Another thing that has a bit less utility, but that helps build rapport and trust, is to speak English the whole time and at the end of the exam ask a question in whatever their language happens to be. It will totally confuse them, because they become so focused on processing your English that they don't even realize you flipped into Chinese or Vietnamese or Thai.

Hell, not only is it fun to do, but in forty years, we will probably figure out it has medical use. Joking involves a wide variety of neural pathways, so if you have told a joke and the other party understands it, you have completed a very extensive cognition test on everything from their occipital visual cortex to their parietal and frontal motor cortices, as well as the temporal lobe with its hearing centers, just to name a few. Basically, a joke can let you make a somewhat gross assessment of all the five cortices. As always, I am potentially ahead of my time.

But the pilots appreciate it when you show them that you are human, that you are willing to be relaxed with them while explaining to them nuances of your nation's regulatory environment as opposed to their own. Rapport goes a long way.

Most complaints are, of course, going to come from pilots. If you are an AME and have never had a pilot complain to you about the FAA, you either don't do enough medicals or you aren't being very particular about doing your job. A third option of being more empathic and people-oriented than I am, I reject out of hand.

▲ ▲ ▲

Character often requires saying uncomfortable things to people, and the art of doing this is a process learned. One day early on in the kindergarten of my learning process, I had an African-American pilot who hadn't flown in about ten years show up for a flight medical. He was a pretty impressive guy, well-educated and in an important position at a very good company. He was also on a beta-blocker, so I asked him about this.

"Yep," he said. "I have high blood pressure."

"Do you know why your doctor chose a beta-blocker?" The reason for my question was curiosity, as I had been trained that beta-blockers were often more useful in younger Caucasians, whereas diuretics were a more effective first line in the African-American population. Granted, this wasn't a hard, fast rule, but I was looking to assess two things: first, did the pilot know why he was on a beta blocker out of large number of HTN classes to choose from, and second, what was the doctor's thought process if the pilot did know.

Well, the pilot didn't know, so we moved on to the next issue.

At that time, hypertension required labs, three blood-pressure readings at least twenty-four hours apart, and a letter from his physician stating he was stable (if I remember correctly). They may have dropped the lab requirement and dropped the ECG requirement prior to this time. He became concerned because he hadn't had to do this the previous time.

I pointed out to him that his last medical was ten years ago, and he had just said he'd started blood pressure medication this year. He was really concerned that he couldn't get three BP readings in the time needed, so I assured him that I would accept today's reading, a reading from a local EMS facility, and then he could come back to pick up the medical and we would count that reading. So off he went.

Now, the FAA had also just changed rules, stating he only had seven days to get this done, because he was still just a student pilot. I called to verify I was reading this change properly, since he had had a previous exam. The AMCD flight doctor assured me that I had to transmit in seven days.

Seven days went by, and the phone rings. It is the pilot, and I explain that I am out of options. I hadn't heard from him, so I was going to have to submit his exam as a deferral, and he would need to send the FAA his information. He then began the long, drawn-out process of thinking he was in a negotiation, while I (initially patiently) knew he was in a rationalization death spiral. First he said he didn't know if going to the EMS site would suffice. I assured him that I was the one who was tasked with deciding which BP readings could be used, so I was 100 percent sure that I was OK with him doing what I'd told him to do.

Then he said he had talked to another AME who was a personal friend and that that AME told him none of this was necessary. I calmly informed him his friend was wrong and calmly refrained from mentioning that if he was that good a friend, then why hadn't he gone to him in the first place. Then he went back to repeatedly asking me if I was sure that they would be OK with an EMS reading. At this point it was irrelevant anyway, since he didn't have twenty-four hours left on the process, but I continued to assure him, that they (meaning I) would be OK with them (meaning me) accepting the EMS blood pressure readings. After all, as I told him repeatedly, EMS are very good and are competent to a fault, as they are the only personnel in medicine constantly faced with being rechecked, and an EMS who shows up telling the ER doc that a patient has a normal BP when the patient is crashing isn't going to last very long.

So then the whole story began that he had checked with *two* AMEs, and *both* of them had told him this wasn't necessary. At this point—I have no idea how—my patience reached an end, and I less than calmly explained that I didn't give one goddamn about his other AME's opinions anymore than they had called me and asked me for mine. I then told him that this conversation, or illegal coercion masked as wheedling, was at an end. *Slam* went the make-believe desk phone! After all, he'd talked, whined, and coerced me for so long that I really had to go pee.

After a quick pause, I regained a sense of professional decorum and realized I should get the FAA on the phone. I did so, simultaneously e-mailing the pilot and apologizing for being "brusque" but reinforcing the process as it was going to work going forward, no matter how many mythical AME tooth fairies he plucked out of his nethers.

I quickly explained the whole situation to the regional flight surgeon's office, letting them know all the nuances, from the beta-blocker question to the EMS visits but leaving off the bathroom visit. Not ten minutes later, the RFS called back and said, "Yep, you nipped that one in the bud. Good job; we set this guy straight. By the way, he refused to tell us the names of these AMEs, but he does believe you to possibly be a raging Kluxer or something." No good deed. The pilot did e-mail me back to make sure I was corrected on the word *brusque*; he felt the word *rude* was a better description. I let that pass; he has a right to an opinion.

▲ ▲ ▲

So I am telling a pilot how I miss the old desk phones because it isn't as gratifying now to slam the phone down. I missed the visceral nature of putting that exclamation point on a call.

The next week, he showed up with a couple of phones in a bag for me to slam when I need too. We have a ton of great pilots, and that was an awesome one.

▲ ▲ ▲

And then there was the other certified letter incident. This event was the second of two times I heard a pilot utter one particular phrase.

In the first incident, a pilot opened the door to my office and yelled, "Doctor Shewmaker, I am going to stay as far away from you as possible, because I am really sick."

Up to the challenge, I yelled back, "Try your house! Can't get much further away than that!" And after only ten minutes of explaining why I couldn't do his medical that day because he wasn't well, he got the idea pretty clearly, and off he went home.

The second time didn't have nearly the same good outcome. There were a lot of nuances to it that are really fun. It was my very first day back after taking two weeks off to have disc replacement surgery on my neck. After allowing the VA to jerk me around like a ragdoll for five years, I had finally gone to a professional medical group and had my neck cut open.

The orthopedic surgeon wanted me to take six weeks off, but I was convinced that two would be plenty, so two weeks to the day, there I was, in a full neck collar. My vocal cords were still not working well, and neck muscles were still sutured to my skin. So with no voice, a lot of Tylenol, and a stiff neck, I was back at it. I practiced on my son for a couple hours to make sure I was actually able to do my job appropriately. I knew it wasn't going to be easy, so I went light on the scheduling.

So on this particular day, in walked a gentleman for an exam, precisely one minute after I had gotten off the phone with AMCD with only a message stating they were gone for the day. I had also helped a guy with a ton of his own self-induced miscues because he'd ignored my advice, had the wrong testing done, waited too long to do it, and so on. Now this gentleman was finally back to get an exam after I obtained verbal authorization from AMCD, but he had shown up just after they had closed up shop, despite my warning him precisely about this issue. So anyway, I explained this to him and spelled out his options for getting a medical, while he sat on my exam table. Then he blurts out, "Doctor Shewmaker, I am going to stay as far away from you as possible, because I am really sick."

At that, I told him, in the marginal whisper that passed for a voice, "Then you need to leave right now."

He wasn't buying that and began to argue, so I pointed to the door and repeated that he needed to leave immediately. At no time was I able to raise my voice, which for me was clearly the most distressing part of this whole story.

Off he goes for his hour or so drive home during rush hour traffic, so sick that he didn't want his flight doctor to even get close to him, but wanting to fly so much that he wanted his flight doctor to lie and say he examined him, while staying as far away as possible, evidently. Who knows? I did chuckle about the fact he must have spent the entire hour or so driving to my office while he was so sick that he must have been thinking, *Gotta remember to warn Shewmaker, gotta remember to warn Shewmaker, gotta remember to warn Shewmaker*—yet evidently the light bulb of my regular lecturing to all pilots not to come if they are sick just never clicked.

So I forgot all about it and put in his paperwork. He got his medical mailed out by the southern region or AMCD, and then came a certified letter. "Shewmaker, a pilot has accused you of yelling at him, telling him to leave, and refusing to do an exam on him because he had a cold."

That was pretty much the tenor of the letter. I can only imagine the laughter the folks of the FAA were having while writing to one of their AMEs to ask him why he stopped a pilot from utilizing poor judgment. But, I was told to answer within five days and reminded that I could lose my right to do flight medicals. So what could I do?

Gotta sit down and write a letter. This one was easy, of course, but I wasn't about to stoop into using my neck surgery as an excuse. If I could have yelled at the rude guy who came to my office after driving an hour knowing he was way too sick to get his medical and who sat in my lobby exposing two other pilots to illness as well as myself, well, you can pretty much guess, I would have done it.

So why try to apologize for not yelling simply because I wasn't physically able to and would have done it? Instead, I simply wrote that the pilot sat on my table and stated he was so sick that he was warning me not to examine him fully, so I did as he asked me to do and sent him home—even though that wasn't really what he wanted. He really wanted me to ignore his warning that he was too sick to be there and wanted me to simply pass him anyway. And that is the essence of how a pilot will attempt to rope you into his or her fraudulent web.

▲ ▲ ▲

Anyway, I was using bits of this story later as part of my "don't come to the exam sick" spiel to another pilot, and when I got to the part about being accused of yelling at a pilot, the pilot said, "But that's just your thing."

To which I had to reply, "You...complete...me!"

▲ ▲ ▲

Back to my marketing campaign and a way to show you that the FAA is well aware that certain AMEs are a bit (a lot) too lenient (criminal) with how they handle (collude with) the pilots who seek them out.

One day when my office was still in Hobe Sound, I was sitting in the back of a Washington Ritz Carlton conference room, listening to all the very old AMEs around me whine about these overpriced conventions (the convention was free), while I laughed internally about my eighty-dollar-a-night Westin Room a short subway ride away that I had got on Priceline. Truly, sitting behind a gaggle of eighty-year-old AMEs and hearing them complain about computers, Internets, and cotton gins is a highlight of these conventions. I picture myself whining about my clones in another thirty years at a holographic convention in the future.

Suddenly, my ears perked up, because the FAA physician at the podium was talking about how they determine whether an AME is a good AME (like me) or a bad AME (like doctors with a 10 percent deferral rate, or a $400-with-no-real-exam practice).

"How do we tell if an AME is a bad actor? Well, we look at a lot of things. How do they advertise? Do they claim to be fast? Do they claim to be friendly? Do they say that they are pilot oriented? Do they mention their price?"

So I slid out my postcard and put it next to me to show the other AMEs that I was advertising *Fast, Friendly, Pilot-Oriented Physicals, $60*. A marvel of alliteration, I might add. I had mixed feelings, as clearly I was being slandered or libeled by someone who has never owned a practice and who was likely reading off one of my own postcards that a different AME had sent the FAA to try to denigrate me. (Well, it was a plausible explanation, since he basically had mentioned my postcard's contents verbatim, but let's give him a benefit of the doubt. Let's listen some more.)

He continued on: "We also look at how far away people travel to see the flight doctor." And with that, he posts a slide showing five practices—no names, just cities.

LA, Chicago, New York, Atlanta, and Hobe Sound. And next to them was the average distance pilots traveled.

Now I was just starting out there, and had just started getting pilots from flight schools who were from Vietnam, China, Korea, and Nigeria. And there was only one AME in the bustling metropolis of Hobe Sound. Me. So, essentially, the FAA physician was openly slandering me as a bad physician, simply because a flight school called me to complain about their old AME who was refusing to help their pilots if they had a medical problem they needed to clear with the FAA. I was being punished and slandered for getting their information as quickly to the FAA doctors as is appropriate and as the FAA training program teaches AMEs to do.

I am not a big fan of having all of my colleagues sit in a room looking at a slide with Hobe Sound, Florida, on it, while they are all wondering, *Hey, I wonder how many doctors are in that town* (answer: one).

So, the FAA is definitely looking at how to detect poor AMEs; however, I am not at all comfortable with them actually having not the first idea of how easy it is to find a poor AME. After all, it isn't rocket science. See the chapter on SOLUTIONS.

21

Complaints Are a Dime a Dozen and Solutions Are Out of Stock

or, Are You Just Going to Whine, or Are You Going to Buy Something?

THE PROBLEMS INHERENT to flight physicals are, on a relative scale, minor. I have dealt with the USCIS (United States Customs and Immigration Service), and their outright fraudulent actions far too much to ever complain seriously about the fairly consistent, predictable, and protocol-driven, outreach-encouraging group known as the FAA.

To juxtapose, let me tell you about the USCIS. They have a medical examination form as well. That way, physicians can examine immigrants attempting to legally reside in the United States.

The form can be filled out on the computer, but it cannot be submitted that way; you must print it out. Then you make three copies, and you give two sealed copies to the non-US citizen. That person then prances around for several months with an official US document in his or her possession that you should have been able to submit electronically. And then the immigrant turns it in…and if there are any slight issues with the form, instead of e-mailing the doctor at the included e-mail address that is required to fill the form out, USCIS makes the immigrant start all over again, thus wasting USCIS time as well as the immigrant's.

In 2013, the four-page form was replaced by a five-page form. The old form had been expired for several months, and we'd been submitting medicals to USCIS on expired forms, with their blessing. The funny part of that was the old and new forms had the expiration dates listed on them, so the USCIS basically knew they would need a new form in 2011, but somehow was unable to create a new one by the time 2013 rolled around. Especially comical is that when the new forms came out they had no substantive changes. They moved some words, added space, made the form five pages long so that they could waste more paper—but the actual information wasn't substantively different. In business we call this stupidity.

On the top left upper part of the page, the new forms stated: "EXPIRES JAN. 31, 2015. So, in March or April of 2013, USCIS was well aware they would need a new form by January 2015.

On January 31, 2015, however, the USCIS once again seemed to have no protocol to bridge its expired forms, so it again openly admitted incompetence and on its website stated (not verbatim): "We can't make a new form yet, so keep using the old form, and we will accept it."

(That's close, except they took no responsibility for their own lack of competency, other than that it was obvious if you were paying attention closely.)

Another important item to realize is that immigration medicals are good for one year from the date the doctors complete them, sign them, and put them in sealed envelopes for non-US citizens to walk around the earth with until such time as the immigration folks decide to have the immigrants send or bring them to them.

This early Sumerian methodology of ignoring modern computers is made more funny by the fact that on the 2013 and new 2015 forms (they finally made one) the USCIS asks for the doctor's e-mail.

Yet in eight years, they have never once used this e-mail to contact us to see if one of the boxes is checked correctly. Instead, they will cancel a person's exam. For example, despite the person being forty and the immigrant official knowing full well that they don't need an Hib vaccination, they will send that person back to the immigration doctor to fix an unmarked box that was staggered somewhere in the massive jumble of incompetent form design. Thus, they waste the immigrant's time, the doctor's time, and their own time by not using common sense and a twenty-first-century solution.

But it gets worse.

When the poor immigrant comes to your office, he or she sees an immigration doctor using expired forms and needs to be consoled that it's OK. We know the form is expired, but the US government told us to use them.

When the new 2015 form finally showed up with its 2017 expiration date, the immigrants received letters stating that the forms they had submitted were old, expired forms, even though at the date of the exam, the form was the only one in existence, and the medical was good for one year. In other words,

1. the USCIS told the immigrants to use the expired form;
2. the USCIS then REFUSED to accept it;
3. the USCIS BLAMED the doctors for using an expired form;
4. the form used was the only one available, due to the incompetency of the USCIS; and
5. the information on the two forms was, for all practical purposes, identical.

This is beyond dishonest; it is sleazy. They made no apology for it being their issue. Thus, the immigrant believes the physician was the dishonest person. So the applicant then has to take off of work again and lose money, so they are upset. And upset immigrants walk in to doctor's offices speaking Vietnamese or Mayan or Farsi or Spanish or German at extremely impressive speeds.

The physician has to deal with random people walking into their lobby ticked off and wanting immediate help, so the physician's staff is ticked off. And this is all so that a nine-page form that is identical in real utility to the previous five-page form can be put into a computer program, and then printed instead of electronically transmitted.

The only change in the new form, which you can view at uscis.gov/i-693, is that it is now nine pages. Layout has made the pages more difficult to use while only adding a page for a translator so that people can certify that their name, date of birth, address, and place of birth are correct. This is likely the only information an immigrant never needed a translator for, because who doesn't know their own address, name, and date and place of birth?

It is a pathetic waste of twenty-seven pages (triplicate) in a time when we are pretending to care about the environment. We have online systems now that could stop a non-US citizen from having to walk the streets with a sealed package of nonsense.

So, let's be clear: the FAA has a very modern, approachable, and important medical system in place. The solutions it needs in my opinion are minor and could be done quickly. So, to the FAA, I would suggest:

1. Look at an AME's rate of deferral and compare it to their phone records to FAA facilities. If they have a high deferral rate and a low phone rate, they are overdeferring.
2. Look at an AME's rate of deferral and compare it to their phone records. If they have a low deferral rate and a low phone rate, they have a higher risk of going rogue. The way a flight physician gets a low deferral rate is by contacting the FAA for verbal authorization, so if you have a nonexistent deferral rate and you aren't calling the FAA for verbals, you are probably not reporting a hell of a lot of very common issues.
3. Look at each AME's geographic area and compare it to their yearly number of physicals. If they are well established and are doing less than 10 percent of people in their area, then call them and try to figure out why. They may not really care that much about doing FAA exams, and if that's the case, don't keep them.
4. Don't worry about the 50 percent of AMEs who are only doing fifty pilots a year. A pilot a week isn't going to give anyone a good concept of the real issues of aviation medicine. Maybe you need the AME because they are in East Rumpsteak, Texas, with thirty-two pilots a hundred miles from Spaghetti Cove, Oklahoma, but watch these pilots with a bit more care.

Don't worry about the AME. Watch the pilots' exams carefully for red flags, such as being seventy and suddenly off the four meds they were on for years. Or being eighty-two and suddenly getting a new medical after eighteen years.

After all, these AMEs are doing less than a tenth of all the exams being done. You can get more out of e-mailing them suggestions and articles, but you aren't going to make huge improvements by focusing on them when your money is on the busy docs.

5. Have a training program to put FAA doctors into busy AME doctor's offices for one or two weeks a year and rotate which offices you show up to. A good AME is one who wants to ensure he or she is complying with what is expected rather than what they have sort of fallen into out of habit without real oversight or input. When you are collegial, you can be corrective; when you are detached, AMEs are simply going to do things the way they think things should be done, and bad habits will form. I would say this is likely ubiquitous to the AME community.

6. Utilize the experience with the AMEs to build a deeper rapport and a source for collaborative and positive change.

7. Slowly cull the AME group to the busiest pilot-oriented group that has a track record of low deferrals combined with collaborative interactions and who aren't openly price gouging the pilot population and then dumping pilots as problems arise. If an AME really is blasé about doing aviation medicals, then they aren't going to mind if you are blasé about keeping him or her around.

8. Get the EMR modernized, seek input from the busiest AMEs for at least six months prior to making any type of change, and assess its impact. This is because large changes can cause attitudes to sour, and when an attitude sours in a person who doesn't feel appreciated or listened to, you are setting the stage for AMEs to simply go rogue.

After all, if you have a hundred AMEs doing two thousand exams a year, you have 33 percent of all pilots at minimum being handled by these one hundred examiners. This makes your oversight and collaborative issues better, and you have economic skin in the game by the AME. These are your people, and they are the ones to nurture.

These eight points are also part and parcel of why we do have bad AMEs and why we haven't figured out how to identify them. You can't sit in a cubicle and use statistics on geographical distance or your total lack of understanding of good marketing and advertising to actually assess the character of an AME. I should know—I was a victim of that false, inane concept of how to make bad decisions by making bad assumptions.

As for pilots and medical issues, there are several things that would improve flight safety fairly quickly. This is off the cuff and far from a comprehensive set of changes. It's also colored with the biases of an AME who is still mad that you haven't voted me king yet.

1. Biannual skills testing and sponsored volunteer and quarterly fitness/skills testing rodeos and contests with rewards, designed to find cognitive deficits and deficits in organization and judgment while educating, brings ideas forward and instills more esprit de corps across the real aviation community than the leeches who pretend to be advancing it.
2. Instead of simply a biennial flight review, pilots who have difficulty with the skills and competency testing should then be aggressively screened for both cognitive and medical issues.
3. A computerized testing of skills and task acquisition and memory retention would also be of great benefit.
4. An anonymous survey as well as investigations to eliminate dangerous pilots from each FBO, each ramp, each field, and each place where they are embarrassing the professional pilots who take safety seriously. Every FBO in America is full of pilots who know who the most dangerous person on the field currently is, and at controlled airfields, the ATC personnel certainly do as well. Acting can save lives; not acting almost certainly will take lives.

5. One thing that could catapult aviation medicine past even regular modern medicine would be the installation of training protocols for handheld echocardiography, standardization, training protocols, and implementation of this technology. We need to replace the stethoscope and relegate this oft abused, and oft poorly used relic to the museum that it is headed inevitably toward at some near time anyway. This may sound revolutionary, but in fact, the death of the stethoscope has already occurred; we are simply engaging in medical necrophilia in still embracing it. Maybe waiting for the future isn't as good a concept as being at the tip of the spear of progress. HA1C and fasting blood-sugar finger sticks are also a much better place to be than the archaic and very unproductive urine glucose testing. That procedure has inherent flaws, not the least of which is how much easier it is for a noncompliant, dishonest pilot to game the system, but an HA1C followed by a confirming fasting blood sugar is a lot more difficult to game.
6. Being first in a hard push to place the handheld echocardiogram into the hands of aviation medical professionals would be invaluable both in demonstrating the worth of aviation medical professionals and that they are modern and emerging, rather than old and retiring. Additionally, it would possibly have the added benefit of culling those AMEs we all know have passed their competency peak and are simply using aviation medicine as a way to earn some spare change and pretend a relevance that has been gone for some time. These AMEs are out there—we all know that they are, so I hesitate to call this a dirty little secret, but I don't hesitate to call it shameful. Having a new technology to learn is either exciting or angst generating. I think the AMEs who are excited about such things are likely going to do a very good job in its implementation.
7. Aggressive punishment of people who clearly are misleading examiners and who then have incidents after that fact. In any regulatory endeavor, there must a Torquemada, willing to dip

the heathen into the vat of oil. This oversight doesn't have to be overly broad, but its application should be fair and visible so that there is an incentive both positively and negatively not to try to game the system.

8. Lastly, it is time to stop the charade that aviation governance somehow needs to be hidden from the medical records of pilots who are flying at the largesse of the public, not by any God-given right. Pilots must present their medical records at each exam, and they should certify that these are correct and accurate. If the pilot is over age fifty and hasn't seen a doctor in at least two years, then we should seriously consider that this pilot simply has such little regard for the concept of preventative maintenance that perhaps the pilot doesn't need to be endangering the public. Obviously, this should be based upon science and best practices; however, we shouldn't pretend that in the case of aviation the rights of a person to have a hobby should somehow be elevated above the rights of the homeowners he elevates his plane over. At some point, it would behoove the aviation medical community to put again to the forefront the concept that above all else we are placed in our positions to protect the safety of the general public, not to protect incompetent folks with diminished skill sets who feel that competency isn't required when arrogance would suffice.

And for those that say this might be the death of general aviation, I would say that for many pilots who have moved outside of their competency levels and a great many aggressive pilots with poor judgment, the cause of the death of general aviation is themselves and often ironically is the cause of their own death as well.

22

Obesity: The Weighty Issue Plaguing America

or, Exercise Is the Cure to Rationalization

When we start to talk about decline of competency, attention to detail, mental acuity, motivation, health, self-esteem, and so on, we have to discuss the most massive issue facing American pilots, as well as FAA personnel and AMEs.

Obesity is a huge problem.

About ten years ago, I got a bit tired and evidently lost my will to chew. With time, I slowly shrank eighty pounds. The entire process took about seven months and was relatively simple, because at the end of the day, losing weight is a matter of *not* doing something. I am an expert at procrastination, so I simply procrastinated my large meals for seven months. It was extremely simple, but it was done with a bit more insight than I am pretending.

1. I figured out that my metabolic daily caloric requirement was about three thousand calories, as I wasn't really exercising a lot.
2. I knew that if I divided my meals up into five or six small meal events per day that I would never be more than an hour away from either just having eaten or just about to eat, so mentally, I wasn't going to be going long periods without food.

3. I shopped only in small daily amounts and with foods that were easy to calorie check. Portioned meats, fruits, vegetable, or packaged items (such as ice cream bars...yep, I ate them like crazy, but I knew the exact calories that should be in them).
4. I limited myself to twenty-five hundred calories, and off came the weight.

About forty pounds into my weight-loss journey, I was driving home with my son in the passenger seat when all of a sudden, I felt a strong, knifelike pain in my upper abdomen. I had no idea what this pain was, but it was significant enough that if the traffic wasn't so light, I'd have immediately pulled over. My son, who was watching me, worried for about a minute and said, "Let's pull into Publix, maybe you just need some Sprite." And on went the lightbulb, and I began to laugh, to the point that my son became worried:

"What, what, what?"

I turned slowly to him. "I know what this is," I said with my best, arrogant, know-it-all, doctor face.

"What, what, what?"

"I am having hunger pains!" I said. And then the second knife hit.

My son said, "Well, now you know how I feel when I tell you I'm hungry and you say, 'OK, we'll eat in a little bit.'"

Children just have a way of making you realize that your mythology of being a great parent sometimes doesn't fit the reality.

After about forty pounds, I had to shift down to two thousand calories because I still hadn't started an aerobic conditioning plan—mainly because I was procrastinating, but I had some great rationalizations about it. So then the other forty pounds came off, and there I was at 170 pounds. Thus, the advocacy of weight loss and the ease at which people could lose weight became a central part of my office theme.

Weight loss usually begins when a person decides to tell the inner voices to shut the hell up. It is only this repetitive internal dialogue that starts the process. The success of the process and its longevity is in the planning and implementation, but all weight loss begins with the following sentence: "That's crap, and I am doing this," or some such tiny voice responding to the best-trained, most professional enemy we have: our inner negative voice.

Over the past twelve years, I have listened to more rationalizations than the entire number of postwar German civilians pretending no culpability in the genocide. It is a gift of humankind that we can create an internal myth of who we are simply by imagining our own reality and ignoring the objective reality that surrounds us. Truly, we are all just bubbles of myth floating around, waiting on the sharp tines of reality to burst our fairy tale. We see it in all things: aging Lotharios, fading A-list actresses disappearing instead of moving to character roles, barstool ex-athletes, and theoretical physicists who suddenly become experts on world affairs, despite being far too naïve to understand the most basic human emotions of jealousy and avarice.

The myths that people create to excuse their obesity are numerous.

- "I'm not that big compared to other people." You need to leave America and travel for six months, because you are a salmon, looking at other big fat salmon, when the rest of the 6.7 billion people on the planet outside of the spoiled, engorged North American continent are mostly perch (thinner).
- "My wife cooks me large meals."
- "I travel too much."
- "I don't have time to exercise."
- "I am home a lot."
- "It's hard to lose weight."
- "I have a slow metabolism."
- "I am big boned."
- "All my family is fat."

Whatever myth you want to create, someone much larger than you has already spewed its falseness into my face amid a cloud of oyster-cracker dust and diabetic breath.

The truth is that these are all nonsense. They are an internal dialogue people use intentionally to prevent themselves from taking action.

The intent is to gain respite from an outside attacking world, and to prop up the walls of their mythological bubble world that defines the narrative of their false reality.

Hell, these mostly ashamed people have even come up with a false narrative called "fat shaming" to try to keep the thorns of reality from bursting into their own world and destroying their self-created, self-defeating, internal dialogue. But it is all just garbage.

Weight loss is easy, but it requires being honest with yourself. If you can't be honest with yourself, then hey, you are not going to succeed. If you can't be honest with yourself, you also need to know that everyone else already knows you aren't being honest with yourself. Your children know it; your family knows it; and you yourself know it, as do your colleagues and friends. If their pointing out a true reality to you shames you, then that isn't their issue, it is your own.

Now, ask yourself a basic question: if weight loss were hard, why would so many companies exist to try to sell you their weight-loss plans? I haven't seen any advertisements on national media telling me that for ten dollars a month someone will teach me to climb Mount Everest, or for twenty-nine dollars a month, someone else will teach me to wrestle a grizzly bear.

Hard things to do don't have a lot of companies offering services; only easy things have a companies offering services. Weight loss, meal planning, exercise, online education. You can lose weight on your own, meal plan on your own, exercise on your own, and learn how to do Excel on your own. But the numbers of companies offering you a hand at it are innumerable. This is a direct ratio to how easy it is to do the thing they are trying to convince you that you need them for. It isn't always the case, but in the self-improvement market, it sure as hell is.

Weight loss is as easy as having a friend lock you in a closet for a month and put a tube under the door, through which you'll suck water and nutrients that they control. In other words, even the craziest weight loss plan will work, provided it matches the basic tenets of physics.

In fact, I'd wager that most weight-loss plans have proven to be wildly successful…the inventors of the gimmick-of-the-week-plans seem to always end up in a nicer house. Thus, all diet plans work, because dieting is simple.

Regardless of metabolism or any other issue, a person who burns three thousand calories per day but only eats twenty-five hundred calories a day will lose weight that day. And I can tell you the amount of weight that day will be one-seventh of a pound, approximately. Thus, a person who every day eats five hundred calories less than what they burn that day will lose fifty-two pounds per year.

That isn't rocket science, but it is basic physics.

So having lost weight and become an advocate lot for weight loss, I quickly learned that helping everyone else with this simple process was a bit more difficult. Losing weight isn't difficult, but breaking down a person's self-rationalization—now there is a task worthy of growing out your hair and pushing apart the pillars of a temple.

My personal history of weight-loss counseling to patients has evolved over time.

First I tried the long lectures. Usually when met with a blank stare, I'd work even harder. Yet, six months or a year later, the pilot would come back, and I'd ask, "Did you lose weight?"

"Nope, but I didn't gain any!"

Thunk, thunk, thunk.

So you are still unhealthy, and you have let one more year slip by on your goal to really bad health? Got it.

Occasionally, I'd hear, "I am down ten pounds." And I'd look at their old medical and find they had actually gained ten pounds.

"But I see here, you actually gained ten pounds."

"Well, yeah. I gained twenty, but I have since lost ten."

Thunk, thunk, thunk.

Sometimes I'd try the harsh, in-your-face approach. This would actually work better than the lecture. I had a gentleman come in who weighed 220 pounds, and six months later a thin guy comes in and I said, "Who are you?"

He said, "I've been here before."

So, I asked him for his driver's license and saw a very obese face staring at me in the photo.

"Tom Morton" [made up name].

"This isn't you; this guy is Tom Morton."

"Yep, it is. I am Tom Morton. I lost eighty pounds in the past six months."

I was curious about his technique so I asked, "How'd you do that, Tom?"

"Well, six months ago, you said either I could be forty-five in ten years and in the best shape of my life, or I could be dead or on my third heart attack. I got scared, so I started bicycling."

"Evidently, you haven't stopped bicycling long enough to eat, Tom."

▲ ▲ ▲

Another gentleman said I did the same thing for him, but that it was both my talk and his divorce that motivated him. He went from looking like the typical American backyard hamburger grill master to looking like a well-balanced, undrugged Lance Armstrong or Greg LeMond. Again, through bicycling. He increased his metabolism. It's simple physics. He wasn't overeating, he was underworking.

▲ ▲ ▲

A couple of months after Tom lost his weight, a gentleman walked in for a flight exam. I started on the exam, getting the past medical history. Suddenly the pilot stopped me by taking hold of my arm. "Wait, my boss, Bob Sanders [made up name], wanted to say thanks for what you did with Tom."

Being a highly intelligent guy, I went bilingual: "Huh?" which is Spanish for "¿que?"

"You know, Tom Morton, the guy that lost all the weight."

"Oh, no problem."

He grabbed hold of my arm once more. "I don't think you understand. Bob really wants to tell you thanks for what you did with Tom."

"OK, so what is the story?" I caught on eventually that there was a bit more conversation in this pilot that had to come out.

"Bob said to tell you that his office has a staff of forty people, and that Tom is his assistant. Once Tom lost all of his weight, the entire office became more motivated, more organized, happier, more cohesive, and more health conscious."

And to this day, it does give me goosebumps, because so much of the time we know we are making a hypothetical impact, but we rarely see the rippling effect of our good deeds, only the repercussions of our sins.

I like that; it is now trademarked.

Well, Tom and his karma just wouldn't let me go, but it did stoke my ego. Renewed, I set about to counsel, work, plead, cajole, and harangue (that's all the synonyms I've got, so we'll move on) pilots to lose weight.

One day, I decided I was going to take a four-day trip to Costa Rica, just to rent a car, drive around, relax, and have an experience outside of my office. And if you are thinking that is code for playing poker, blackjack, and climbing volcanos, you might be close as well. Costa Rica had changed in the twenty years since I had last visited, and I realized two things quickly. They had discovered the car, and they had not discovered driving instruction. I also learned that when asked if you want a GPS in Costa Rica, there is only one correct answer to this question. It is not a yes or no question; it is a *yes, period,* question. I call their signage early American garage sale, because you may turn left at one sign, then right at the next, but ten minutes later when you come to a fork in the road, there isn't a sign, and you have no idea if the garage sale (or volcano, in this case) is to the left or right. One intersection was a lot easier though: I came to a stop sign; the road turned left, and the road turned right. And right there at the stop sign was a sign that said: VOLCANO, and the two arrows on it pointed, one left and one right.

Anyway, as I boarded the airplane, I saw Tom Morton and his wife on the plane as well. In fact, they were one seat in front of me in the other aisle with a group of their friends. I had never met Tom's wife. Tom offered me all kinds of free drinks, but I am not a big alcohol drinker, so I settled on water and sat back to head to San Jose, hoping the pilots knew the way and that an AME who was competent had done their latest flight exams. Midway through the flight, Tom's wife leaned over across him and looked directly back at me, which temporarily startled me as I was reading my *SkyMall* magazine and wondering whether to buy the Egyptian mummy/bar or the ogre coming out of the quicksand.

"I just wanted to tell you thank you for saving my husband's life," she said.

▲ ▲ ▲

And if that isn't enough of a story, about two years later, another incident occurred that really showed the ripple effect a person can have when he or she decides to throw just a little pebble into the pond.

A pilot came into my office and very proudly stated, "I lost forty-five pounds this year!"

Now, I like to be praised as much as the next person, so I baited him with, "Wow, good job! What did I say that had such an impact?"

"Oh, you didn't really say anything."

Grumbling because I just knew I had been the cause of this pilot's sudden change in life and he was denying me my fair due, I went about my business. When I ran out of under-the-breath-grumbling-and-cursing vocabulary a few minutes later, I said, "So, how did you lose the weight?"

He said to me, "Well, it's a bit of a strange story. I was headed into San Juan, Puerto Rico, for a night on the town, and we were in this really nice hotel. As I was going past the hotel gym, I ran across a guy who was a mentor to me when I first started flying. I hadn't seen him for a couple of years, and I hardly recognized him. He was really thin, so I asked if he was OK. And he said, 'Well, about two years ago up in Orlando, I went to get my FAA medical, and the AME looked at me and said: 'You do realize you are going to be forty-five in ten years, right? So, make a choice—are you going to be forty-five and in the best shape or your life, or are you going to have a widow or be on your third heart attack?'"

And with those words, I pointed to the pilot and said, "What was that guy's name?"

And he said, "Tom Morton."

I still get goose bumps typing that.

I pointed my finger into his chest and said, "How dare you try to deny me my secondary ripple effect, you ungrateful son of a radish!"

And for the smallest amount of time, he may have thought, *This AME has lost his mind!*

But we got it all straightened out. Hopefully.

Since that time, I have mellowed the technique a little bit. I am not sure whether it is just part of my nature to get excited about a topic and then, once I have had success, move on to something else, or whether the new technique works. What I do now, though, is ask the pilot, "So, what do *you* think is your largest health issue?" Then I let the pilot tell me that his or her weight is a huge issue. This gives me power to point out that I did not bring it up; he or she did. That makes me the collaborator in fixing the issue instead of a condemning inquisitor.

And with that, I feel I have succeeded in this book and am going to move on to other things now. Thanks for reading. It is greatly appreciated.

23

Bad Judgment Is a Medical Diagnosis

or, Many Pilots Live in a Veritable Fog of Made-up "Facts"

SOME SERIOUS THINGS to consider after reflecting upon these anecdotes. These anecdotes exist within a larger framework. A system is in place to hopefully increase safety in aviation, which some would like to relax. They wish to relax this system because of their belief in falsehoods and fairytales. While myths and silliness may make for good reading in a book on anecdotes, when it comes to aviation, myths and silliness can kill innocent lives.

One such silliness perpetuated by a total lack of insight into aviation accident investigations has been that medically caused accidents are very rare and comprise only 1 to 2 percent of all fatal accidents. This is total nonsense.

It happens because of a basic misunderstanding of English, science, and physiology, as well as a lack of understanding that the human brain is a part of medicine.

One of the main issues is that there are not a lot of solid scientific studies on fatal accidents and their antecedent factors. Thousands of innocent passengers have been killed in fatal GA accidents. Having a real solid handle on how many of these accidents have medical factors that contributed to the fatal accident occurring would be invaluable.

With this in mind, I performed two studies. One study involved light-sport accidents, and the other study involved GA fatal accidents. It is abundantly clear based upon these two studies that medical causes are involved in well over one-third of all fatal aviation accidents and plausibly in over 50 percent of them. I have included these two studies here.

I researched all fatal accidents in the United States during the past fifteen years that involved the most prevalent and ubiquitous airframe, the Cessna 172.

Since its inception, about forty-three thousand units in various configurations of the 172 have been made, and there have been approximately 1,640 fatal accidents with approximately seventeen hundred passengers killed. For the memories of these innocent persons, it is imperative one attempt to get some sense of the real causes of aviation fatalities.

If you extrapolate this to all fatal accidents in GA, one would surmise the number of innocent victims would range at about eighteen thousand. To put that into real perspective, if you look at the number of reported deaths from hurricanes, floods, rip currents, tornados, heat, cold, and lightning strikes in the United States since 1940, you are at about sixteen thousand deaths (source: NOAA).

The usefulness of the Cessna 172 in studying such accidents is abundantly clear when we look at its use and utility. It is a primary trainer, a workhorse utility aircraft, a low-cost, entry-level platform for new airplane owners, and an extremely common rental unit.

It is the most mass-produced platform in general aviation. Thus, using its statistics regarding accident fatalities that are nonmechanical and that involve medical or judgment issues will likely transfer to all other platforms. This is with the caveat that using the 172 as an example platform may actually cause an underreporting of medical causes of accidents, as a person with medical issues will have a more difficult time with a more complex airframe.

In other words, as the complexity of the airframe increases, the risk of poor judgment and medical disqualifications increasing the risk to the airframe should logically be expected to increase. Therefore, one should consider the Cessna 172 data a floor for medical causes of aviation accidents rather than a ceiling.

There have been 252 fatal accidents in Cessna 172s mentioned in the NTSB database since January 2000 that occurred in the United States and for which the NTSB has completed factual and final probable cause reports. I researched the NTSB data and found that almost never did the NTSB pull all the pilot's former medical records from the pilot's personal doctor, or better yet, his or her insurance-billed medical problems. This also means that for many of the accidents that haven't been assigned a medical cause, we can predict that a medical problem might also have been causative, however this is only a very likely probability, versus a known fact. It is clear from reading the basic information that NTSB does report that at least 40 percent of these fatal accidents have probably been medically related.

The number of definitely medical-related accidents puts to rest the completely mythological conjecture that few fatal GA accidents are medically related. It begs the question, how did this myth come to be?

The truth is likely related to how the NTSB determines accident causality. Their very conservative nature in approaching accidents is laudable and appropriate, but it has an unfortunate and predictable byproduct. The NTSB will not call an accident medically caused without very compelling evidence that incapacitation occurred at the moment of either impact or loss of control. But clear and compelling evidence rarely exists in a burned corpse within a burned airframe. Furthermore, sudden and complete incapacitation is only one aspect of medical impairment. If you wreck an airplane due to a slowly developing incapacitation or a partial incapacitation, you are still dead and the cause was still a medical cause. It's common sense, and surprisingly (sarcasm) the people pushing for doing away with the aviation medical examination seem not to grasp this point.

The reluctance of NTSB to call many accidents medically caused has allowed people who perhaps are a bit less literate, trained, intelligent, or who have an agenda, to surmise that since NTSB wouldn't call an accident medical, then it must not have been medical. This is patently silly, because finding a dead corpse without any remaining organs doesn't mean the corpse was organless.

To combat the blatant misrepresentation and even dishonesty of claiming there are few medically related accidents, we can simply look at the NTSB database and read the factual reports. We would discover that a great many fatal GA accidents are not only medically related, they are clearly medically related. It is also clear that we can assume many of the unclear accidents are also medical, but for the sake of discussion we will first start with a baseline using only the clearly medical-related accidents

To determine if a fatal Cessna 172 accident was medical or not, I used several criteria that the reader is welcome to argue with, accept, or modify, as I have posted a list of every single NTSB reported Cessna 172 fatal accident, to which I assigned a medical probability in the appendix. A scale of one to five, rating the severity of the medical issue/judgment was devised, wherein a ranking of three or higher indicated clear and obvious medical impairment, and under three was more probable than proven.

I then asked the following question for each flight: given the information, medication, judgment, training, mental abilities, and so on, would a properly trained pilot with good judgment have turned the ignition on that aircraft for that flight that day?

Out of 229 fatal accidents in Cessna 172 airframes within the past sixteen years with a completed final NTSB report, fifteen of these accidents were almost certainly suicides. In other words, simply looking at the mental health aspect of a severely depressed individual deciding to kill themselves, 6.5 percent of all twenty-first century Cessna 172 fatal accidents were likely suicides. It wouldn't be unreasonable to put an additional 3 percent into that mix, due to the number of crashes (over one hundred) wherein a clear cause couldn't be found.

It is with almost 100 percent certainty that one can surmise that 5 to 10 percent of all general aviation fatal accidents are suicide, if we accept the premise that a Cessna 172 is an excellent marker of overall general aviation, if not a conservative measure due to its excellent operational ease of use.

Thus, before we look at all other crashes, we must start with the premise that 5 to 10 percent of all fatal crashes were likely suicides. All of these crashes are medical causative crashes, as mental health pretty clearly is a medical condition. Hopefully, no one will be crazy enough to argue otherwise.

What other criteria can we use? A clear pattern of sociopathic behavior that resulted in the pilot flying on the day that they crashed when a sane, rational person would have realized they shouldn't be flying. Use of a sedating medication that the FAA has told pilots not to fly while using is another. Other medical causes would be the sociopathic use of illegal narcotics or the illegal flight of the drunken pilot. These are all medical crashes, as the pilot clearly was flying illegally, whether by choice or bad judgment, and the result was that they died. This is fairly well the definition of sociopathic behavior: when one's narcissistic arrogance places them into a situation from which they are at odds with society and that has a negative impact upon their life, in this case, quite literally.

These crashes, however, have varying degrees with which a reader might assume the pilot's decision making showed evidence of impairment; thus, I have devised a one-to-five rating, and placed each fatal accident into a category based upon the number of decisions the pilot made before the flight that were clearly decisions a rational person would be expected not to make. A person who was taking methamphetamine might be given a level five, whereas a gentleman who maybe was doing some low-level flying without recent experience who then hit power lines might warrant a one or a two.

Using this ranking criteria, the following crashes are listed that I have determined are either clearly medical (ranking three to five), strongly probable medical (ranking two), and probable medical (ranking one). I encourage you to read the accident reports and decide for yourself a different criterion.

The results of my study are as follows.

Out of 229 twenty-first-century fatal Cessna 172 accidents, 111 were probably medically related. In seventy-nine of these accidents, there were clear medical reasons why the pilot shouldn't have flown the airplane on the day that they flew. This means that we can predict judgment and medical fatal accidents in general aviation to be definitively above 33 percent, probably at least 48.5 percent, and likely a good 10 percent higher than that yet, due to a lack of data on many of the other fatal accidents. After all, in many accidents the NTSB wasn't able to glean strong medical information regarding either the existence or the absence of a known condition, either due to lack of adequate cadaver material for sampling, lack of a body altogether, or a paucity of past medical records to review.

This relates then that well over half of all fatal general aviation accidents are likely medically related, and thus the clearly erroneous concept that medical issues aren't usually related to aircraft accidents can be pretty soundly put to bed.

We additionally may need stronger mental health screenings, as well as more constancy in reminding pilots not to fly on narcotics or sedating antihistamines. Alcohol, sedating medications, or marijuana were found at significant levels in 14 percent of the fatal accidents. This means that excluding all other fatal accident causes, suicides or medications that were illegal or sedating drugs are found 20 percent of the time. This part isn't conjecture or arguable; it is the actual finding. 20 percent of all fatal Cessna 172 accidents involved sedatives and/or probable suicide.

Thus, the idea that medical causes are rare in fatal GA accidents, when in fact, they occur upward of 50 percent of the time, is not just a myth, it is patently and recklessly not true.

As discussed in the next study, this has an added interesting byproduct. Since it is now clear that approximately half of all general aviation accidents are likely medically or mentally/judgment related, we can now say that for safe pilots who aren't utilizing poor judgment, aviation is far safer than what we were previously assuming. It is the diseased, mentally ill, drugged, or frankly stupid pilots who are causing approximately 50 percent of all fatal accidents. Prior to this study, the mythology was that these diseased, mentally ill, drugged, and frankly stupid pilots were only causing 1.5 percent of fatal accidents. This study shows that for competent, healthy pilots, fatal accidents occur far less often than formerly believed.

A fleshed out discussion of this study and how I determined which accidents were medical or not medical is in my next book, *Murder in a 172*.

TABLE OF CESSNA 172 FATAL ACCIDENTS THAT I HAVE CATEGORIZED AS MEDICALLY RELATED, 2000-2016 time frame:

Incident	year	rank	incident	year	rank
WPR13FA116	2013	1	MIA01FA163	2001	3
ERA13LA281	2013	1	SEA03FA013	2002	3
NYC00FA257	2000	1	DEN02FA084	2002	3
DEN00FA149	2000	1	CHI03LA216	2003	3
NYC02FA012	2001	1	CHI03FA151	2003	3
FTW03FA053	2002	1	MIA03FA066	2003	3
MIA03FA124A	2003	1	IAD05LA028	2004	3
LAX05LA073	2005	1	NYC05LA033	2004	3
NYC06FA154	2006	1	ATL04FA130	2004	3
ERA09FA092	2008	1	LAX06LA064	2005	3
WPR10LA307	2010	1	CHI06LA005	2005	3
ERA11FA493	2011	1	MIA05FA140	2005	3
WPR11FA242	2011	1	DFW05FA082	2005	3
CEN14FA453	2014	1	DFW07FA019	2006	3
CHI03FA071	2003	2	NYC06FA104	2006	3
CEN14FA453	2014	2	CHI07FA140A	2007	3
NYC00FA112	2000	2	ERA09LA132	2009	3
LAX01FA129	2001	2	ERA10LA233	2010	3
LAX01FA070	2001	2	ERA10FA202	2010	3
SEA02FA125	2002	2	ERA13FA388	2013	3
ATL03FA142	2003	2	WPR13FA116	2013	3
SEA05FA013	2004	2	ERA12FA483	2012	3
IAD04FA031	2004	2	WPR12FA274	2012	3
DEN04FA104	2004	2	WPR12FA105	2012	3
ATL04FA099	2004	2	CHI03FA086	2003	4
LAX06FA059	2005	2	DEN01FA028	2000	4
NYC06FA071	2006	2	LAX01FAMS01	2001	4
LAX08FA256	2008	2	CHI03FA086	2003	4

Incident	year	rank	incident	year	rank
LAX08LA191	2008	2	LAX04FA096	2004	4
CHI08LA101	2008	2	DFW07FA049	2007	4
ERA09LA527	2009	2	ERA10FA091	2009	4
ERA10LA105	2010	2	CEN11LA138	2011	4
CEN12LA059	2011	2	LAX03FA109	2003	5
ERA14LA346	2014	2	MIA03FA066	2003	5
ERA12FA193	2012	2	LAX03FA100	2003	5
ANC00FA110	2000	5	CEN12FA154	2012	5
ANC00FA082	2000	5	WPR12LA093	2012	5
LAX01LA286	2001	5	CEN13FA012	2012	5
NYC01FA147	2001	5	ERA12LA578	2012	5
CHI01FA064	2001	5	ERA12FA572	2012	5
MIA02FA104	2002	5	WPR12FA230	2012	5
DEN02FA017	2002	5	SEA05FA125	2005	5
ATL02FA032	2002	5	CHI06FA184	2006	5
LAX04LA089	2003	5	CHI06LA070	2006	5
FTW04FA045	2003	5	LAX08FA023	2007	5
FTW03FA184	2003	5	WPR09LA056	2008	5
LAX03FA109	2003	5	DEN08FA155	2008	5
SEA04FA191	2004	5	LAX08FA261	2008	5
LAX04FA291	2004	5	DFW08FA078	2008	5
ERA14LA084	2004	5	WPR09LA149	2009	5
ANC14FA002	2013	5	CEN10FA101	2010	5
NYC06FA025A	2005	5	ERA11FA369	2011	5
MIA05LA158	2005	5	WPR11FA241	2011	5
NYC05FA138	2005	5	WPR14FA078	2013	5
CHI05FA194	2005	5	ERA14FA027	2013	5
			ERA13FA330	2013	5

To read an NTSB report, you can highlight the id number and put it into a google search. I encourage you to do so and to do your own analysis.

24

Retrospective Assessment of Medical Factors and Decision-Making in Light-Sport Aircraft Fatal Accidents

or, Why Incapacitation Is Hardly the Real Measure of Whether an Accident Is Medically Related

Abstract:

A DEARTH OF INFORMATION coupled with a plethora of misinformation exists involving the role of medical factors in light-sport aviation. Because of the lack of quality information related to medical roles in light-sport fatalities, this study looks at the relationship between medical issues, decision-making, judgment, and aircraft fatalities. The data set only included accidents where toxicological assessment and/or medical records were included in the NTSB findings.

Methodology:

I first did a search of the NTSB aviation accident database, using the parameters: General Aviation, Fatal, "light sport," in the appropriate limit fields.

This netted a total number of 146 accidents. Of these 146, ones in which a probable cause finding had been completed by the NTSB resulted in a total number of accidents of 136.

I then sorted the accidents into two sets.

Set one. The NTSB included medical and toxicological information.

Set two. The NTSB either couldn't do this type of assay due to the severity of victims' burns/decomposition, or the reports simply didn't mention toxicology or autopsy findings.

This left a final data set of 121 fatal accidents. I then reviewed all of these accidents and asked a very simple set of questions from a medical/psychological point of view.

1. Were there preexisting medical conditions that the pilot should have been aware of and that would have made a reasonable physician with integral knowledge of the judgment, training, health, and cognitive skills necessary to fly an airplane have advised that pilot not to fly, and would have a reasonable pilot having asked for such advice, still have flown that day?

2. Were there conditions of weather, training, or even fatigue that would have made a reasonable person with sane mental status decide not to fly, yet this person chose instead through poor cognitive skills to fly?

If these questions were clearly answered, then this accident was assigned a medically preventable accident, since psychotic or sociopathic behavior outside of the norm and cognitive deficits involving judgment are well-recognized medical conditions.

The final decision I used then is: should that pilot have turned on the ignition or should (due to medical reason or obvious judgment) the pilot not have turned on the ignition? Clearly, this becomes a subjective decision, and thus I have included a listing of every NTSB accident number at the end of this report so that you can do your own subjective research and decide for yourself.

Results:

Of 121 fatal accidents, fifty-two (43 percent) were due to medical reasons or due to such extremely poor judgment as to have rendered the pilot incapable of sane cognition concerning their own safety. This was an extremely conservative estimate, and didn't include several cases wherein the sole reason for possible calling the accident a medically bad decision was a sedating antihistamine; even though, potentially, the underlying condition requiring the antihistamine, such as seasonal allergies, may have been affecting vision, alertness, and judgment.

Discussion:

In this review of 121 fatal accident reports by NTSB, it is clear that over 40 percent of them were preventable by a sane person using good cognition with insight into their own medical conditions and/or the current situation/training/weather. It is also clear that to fully assess aviation medical factors, we need better access to previous records relating to the pilot's health, especially as it would affect their judgment. Cognitive skills are a well-recognized medical parameter, and thus, poor utilization of cognitive skills would be a causative factor if the pilot demonstrated such poor cognition as to have gotten into an aircraft on a day that a rational person with medically intact cognitive skills wouldn't have done so.

When one considers that traditionally, the NTSB only considers incapacitation when assessing medical cause and unfortunately doesn't ask if a reasonable person would have turned on the ignition, this study points to a situation wherein we are grossly underestimating the role of poor health and poor judgment in light-sport fatal accidents. Of additional interest is the possible relationship of the sedating antihistamines and fatal accidents in LSA, as in over 5 percent of all fatal accidents, sedating antihistamines were present during toxicology examination, and as this survey didn't address nonfatal incidents, the role of these medications in other incidents bears closer scrutiny. This may simply be anomalous due to the ubiquitous nature of sedating antihistamines in the human population as a whole.

In the end, if we only look at incapacitation and do not consider whether the pilot's initial decision to get into the aircraft was a reasonable and sane decision, we miss the big picture and do a disservice to the general public and to aviation safety. When AOPA has already reported an accident rate in LSA that is three times higher than that of general aviation, it is perhaps time to use a better measurement of aviation safety than incapacitation when assessing accidents. After all, incapacitation is almost impossible to demonstrate after the fact, if the pilot is deceased and decomposed or has suffered major burns. Reasonableness of decision-making is a much easier parameter to assess.

An interesting side effect of this resetting of the reasons behind fatal accidents exists as well. In the past, when mythology and misinformation led people to believe that very few accidents were medically related, this meant that mechanical and training causes would have been assumed a bigger problem. In fact, when we state with near certainty that nearly half of all fatal LSA accidents are medically and/or mentally related, we then are almost halving the number of crashes we would have formerly placed in other categories.

This would necessarily mean that when a pilot obtains quality training, is not impaired, and has utilized baseline human judgment, aviation is not nearly as dangerous as we formerly would have assumed. For good pilots and their families, this is welcome news, as it should also be to anyone who wishes to understand the real risks of general aviation.

Conclusion:

Medically identifiable factors are a major component in LSA fatal accidents, and in all but one of these fatal accidents (a ruptured berry aneurysm), these conditions would have been identified on an aviation medical examination if the AME had access to the patient's family physician's office notes and their prescription history. An additional factor is that many of these pilots had already been informed by AMEs or the FAA that they were not healthy enough to fly without close monitoring; yet, these pilots chose instead to lapse their medicals and to continue to fly despite having obvious judgment issues. This would indicate a need to tighten medical requirements for pilots rather than to loosen them. It also points to a major flaw in the light-sport regulation that allows people to fly unmonitored when the FAA had already placed them on a special issuance process because the FAA stated openly that they needed closer monitoring. Placating a special interest group despite knowing they posed a greater risk to safety by your own parameters seems more a political decision than a safety decision.

Again, I encourage you to read these reports in detail and come to your own conclusions, as your opinion may vary, but without bothering to read the actual reports you limit your own ability to fully understand the nuances of how the NTSB reports are presented.

TABLE OF NTSB REPORTS REGARDING FATAL LIGHT SPORT ACCIDENTS WITH PROBABLE MEDICAL CAUSATIVE FACTORS.

WPR14FA165	CEN10LA401	ERA11LA056	ATL04LA057	WPR10LA462
CEN10LA526	CEN14LA192	WPR10LA292	WPR13FA376	ERA10LA203
CEN13FA338	ERA10LA164	ERA13FA227	ERA10LA119	ERA13FA219
WPR10LA104	ERA13LA09	WPR09LA453	CEN13FA078	ERA09LA502
CEN13LA063	CEN09LA255	CEN12FA638	ERA09LA15	CEN12LA634
ERA09LA013	WPR12FA295	ANC09FA003	ERA12FA395	MIA08LA164
CEN12LA307	MIA08LA161	CEN12LA203	NYC08LA225	ERA12FA107
NYC08LA165	CEN12FA073	NYC08LA087	ERA12FA006	CHI08LA031
ERA11LA496	LAX08LA024	ERA11FA435	DFW07LA102	ERA11LA427
NYC07FA025	ERA11LA415	LAX07FA026	CEN11FA480	MIA06LA135
CEN11LA421	DEN05FA101			

Epilogue

Is This a Full Stop or Touch and Go?

THIS EPILOGUE IS in many regards an introduction. In my next book, *Death in a 172*, I will break down the exact reasons I determined that, at minimum, 47 percent of all fatal Cessna 172 accidents are medically related when one considers that judgment occurs in the brain. It will be look at the suicides, the narcotics, the antipsychotic-medication-related crashes one by one, and by its end I hope that you will have come to a similar conclusion regarding the need for medical oversight in general aviation.

The book following that one will be called: *Head in the Sand, Death in the Cloud*. It will focus on breaking down the Cirrus and Light Sport fatal accidents and will explore the process by which the NTSB investigates accidents.

This book is the culmination of fourteen years and doesn't reflect an overall assessment of pilots in any way. However, its anecdotes are real; the events actually happened. This is concerning, because as we all are aware, there are a great many members of society who act as if they don't need to follow its rules. This is why we have rules, and thankfully, for most people in society this never becomes an issue. Yet, when a person with no regard for safety is flying over your property, you need to have the same right to know about the truth as they do to utilize your airspace.

Printed in Great Britain
by Amazon